# The Every Day Gourmet

to: June (Bug)

" Make EveryDAy Gourmet "

# The Every Day Gourmet

## Quick and Healthy Recipes from Around the World

*Michael Malkoff*

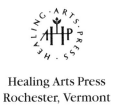

Healing Arts Press
Rochester, Vermont

Healing Arts Press
One Park Street
Rochester, Vermont 05767
Healing Arts Press is a division of Inner Traditions International
www.InnerTraditions.com

*Note to the reader: This book is intended as an informational guide. The remedies, approaches, and techniques described herein are meant to supplement, and not to be a substitute for, professional medical care or treatment. They should not be used to treat a serious ailment without prior consultation with a qualified health care professional.*

Library of Congress Cataloging-in-Publication Data

Malkoff, Michael.
    The every day gourmet : quick and healthy recipes from around the world / Michael Malkoff.
       p.     cm.
    Includes index.
    ISBN 0-89281-785-2 (pbk. : alk. paper)
    1.  Quick and easy cookery.    2.  Cookery (Natural foods)    3.  Cookery,
International.    I.  Title.
TX833.5.M35      1998
641.5'55—dc21                                                     98-41646
                                                                 CIP

Printed and bound in the United States

10 9 8 7 6 5 4 3 2 1

Text design and layout by Kristin Camp
This book was typeset in Garamond and Gill Sans

# CONTENTS

## Soups 15

## Salads 27

## Seafood 89

# Poultry

# Desserts

*For Fredda*

*For Love*

# Preface

I've always described my food as "pretty healthy international favorites that anyone can prepare with minimal time and expertise." It's a mouthful, but it says it all, almost. This is not a macrobiotic cookbook. This is not a vegetarian cookbook. This is not your standard low-fat cookbook. This is my cookbook and I'd like to tell you how it came to be.

In 1983 I stumbled into a macrobiotic restaurant in my neighborhood in Soho. I perused the menu and settled on the macro platter. I was impressed with the "nature" of the food. I felt like I had gone back in time. On my plate there was a connection to the Earth. I became a regular.

This was a starting point for me. From then on, I made my food choices from the ground up. If this sounds strange, well, I guess all transformations do.

I was raised in Ohio where all the food came in packages from the supermarket. Food was a product that was bought and sold. *Grown?* What? I didn't get it. I used to marvel at putting a steak, still in its package, into the microwave, watching it spin around and turn gray through the window. That was food.

Eating grains, beans, vegetables, and seaweed was a grounding experience. It helped me to understand where the food came from and what it was in relation to me as a person. I was a twenty-something macrobiotic.

Around 1987 I began a small business cooking for people in their homes, going into their kitchens and preparing enough food to last for a few days. After the first few months, I got so busy I decided it would make more sense to cook at home and deliver the food to my clients. MMMM Catering was born and I delivered five-course meals twice a week throughout the greater Boston area.

Men and women do not live by brown rice alone (especially when they're paying someone else to be creative). It was a challenge to come up with a different five-course meal two times a week, every week, but my business depended on it. I looked to international cuisine for variety.

Searching the globe for variations on the vegetarian theme reminded me of my love for all sorts of food, including, but not limited to, my nostalgia for junk food, eating off the bone, ceremonial feasts, whatever friends from other cultures put on my plate, and a need to be healthy and connected—in other words, enjoying all of life's offerings.

I began to branch out. I included poultry, seafood, and naturally sweetened desserts in my diet. I continued to abstain from dairy because it didn't agree with my system. I found that it wasn't necessary to eat in health-food restaurants. I saw the world on my plate.

The recipes in this book are the result of my search for the perfect meal. They're real food for real people with discriminating palates and limited time to spend in the kitchen. These recipes cross continents, keep to most of our diets, and won't leave anyone feeling deprived.

I've heard that the whole world, or universe, is within each of us. It's certainly true that the *foods* of the world can be. I hope *The Every Day Gourmet* begins to make it possible. Good eating and good health!

**TIP**

*When buying a cookbook, ask yourself these questions: Are these recipes I would really make? Will I have to turn pages (too complicated) to make a single dish? Do I have the equipment involved? Will it make me an every day gourmet?!*

# Introduction

*The Every Day Gourmet* cookbook is an international guide to well-being. The foundations of most ethnic cuisines are the grains, vegetables, fruits, and protein foods that compose a healthy diet. This book presents simple, healthy, and delicious comfort foods from around the world in an easy-to-use format. It's the multicultural experience that adds mucho variety and international flair to your daily fare.

"I don't have time" and "I'm tired of eating the same thing" are by far the most common complaints that I hear about eating at home. As a chef, I'm very particular about what I eat at home. I want meals to be healthy and interesting without spending too much time in the kitchen. *The Every Day Gourmet* is the result of my search for the perfect everyday meals, "good for you" foods from around the world that make it easy to be healthy

The recipes in this book can be prepared by anyone who can find the kitchen. With few exceptions, the ingredients can be found in most large grocery stores and none of the dishes will take more than an hour to make.

So dig in, have fun, and make the most of food—every day.

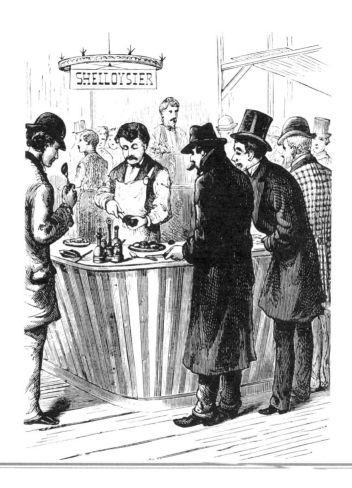

# APPETIZERS

# Homestyle Smoked Salmon Board

*As much fun to make as it is to eat. Homestyle but fancified, if you know what I mean. Cedar wood gives the dish an aromatic accent. Pine is nice too. (Make sure the wood is untreated. Any lumber or hardware store should be able to accommodate you. Wash the board with soap and water and rinse well before using.)*

I pound fresh salmon filet, skin and
   pin bones removed, sliced thin
I tablespoon olive oil
I teaspoon sweetener
Salt and pepper to taste
I package fresh herbs (thyme, dill,
   or cilantro)
3 lemons, sliced very thin

Preheat oven to 350°F. In a small bowl, blend the oil with the sweetener and salt and pepper. Brush an 8 by 12-inch, $^1/_2$- to I-inch thick board with a small amount of the oil mixture and arrange the salmon to cover.

Brush the salmon slices with the remaining oil mixture, cover with the fresh herbs, and lay the lemon slices on top. Bake in preheated oven for 10 minutes and serve hot on the board.

*I tried this Homestyle Smoked Salmon Board on top of the stove, but couldn't keep the board from burning. I'm famous for fires in the kitchen. I remember being a kid and cooking "crackers" over cinder blocks with a match fire—the JD chef strikes again. It's always exciting to have the fire department show up for a cooking class. Cooking essentially combines the element Fire (and sometimes Water) with organic matter, with us chefs as the middlemen. It's primal and delicious.*

# Chili Jicama Sticks

*Jicama is a cross between an apple and a potato. Adding chili southwesternizes this well-bred inbred.*

1 jicama, peeled and cut French-fry
  style
Juice of 2 limes
Pinch of salt
$^1/_2$ to 1 teaspoon chili powder

Lay the jicama on a plate in an attractive manner (always), douse with lime juice, and sprinkle with salt and chili powder. That's it!

*When I'm bored (foodwise or otherwise), I eat ethnic. I seek a splash of culture to transport me to another sensual arena. If I'm really bored, I'll go for something extremely hot and spicy (a chili wake-up call). I agree with Joseph Campbell that what we are all seeking is the experience of being fully alive—I'm just skipping the Upanishads and taking the food route.*

# Salmon Tartare

*Make sure the salmon's absolutely fresh. If there's a Japanese or Korean food store around that sells fish, try it. These guys know what they're doing.*

1 12-ounce fresh salmon filet,
   skinned and boned
1 tablespoon olive oil
2 tablespoons lemon juice
1 clove garlic, finely minced
2 tablespoons chopped parsley
1 tablespoon fresh chopped thyme
   leaves
1 tablespoon capers
Few drops Tabasco sauce
Salt and pepper to taste
2 scallions, finely chopped, as
   garnish
1 teaspoon lemon zest, as garnish

Chop the salmon with a knife into very small chunks.

   Combine all other ingredients (except garnish) in a bowl and add the salmon. Refrigerate for an hour or so.

   Serve in a mound, garnished with scallions, lemon zest, and additional capers if desired.

*I think raw fish is about the most beautiful food on the planet. Super-fresh salmon glistens, it sparkles, it beckons to be consumed. I can almost inhale it.*

   *Sometimes, as a treat, I buy a whole side of salmon. A 3-pound side comes from a 9- to 10-pound fish (almost 40% of the weight of a whole fish is the head, bone, and viscera, leaving in this case approximately 6 pounds of flesh to be divided into two 3-pound sides). Buy one sometime and make a salmon feast (there are four salmon dishes in this book). For a really fishy feast, top the salmon tartare with some rich, red salmon roe.*

# Tempura

*Anything animal or vegetable is fair game for tempura. Slice hard vegetables like carrots and sweet potatoes thin, leave mushrooms whole, cut onions into rings. Serve tempura hot from the pan with its delicious dipping sauce.*

**For the batter:**
1 egg yolk
$^3/_4$ cup ice water (without the ice)
$^3/_4$ cup flour
$^1/_2$ teaspoon salt

**For the dipping sauce:**
$^1/_4$ cup soy sauce
1 tablespoon white wine or sake
1 tablespoon grated ginger
$^1/_4$ cup water
1 teaspoon sweetener
2 scallions, thinly sliced

**You'll also need:**
16 ounces or so peanut or canola
    oil
Assorted vegetables or seafood for
    frying, prepared as desired

Mix the ingredients for the batter together until well blended and put it in the freezer for 10 minutes to chill.

Put peanut or canola oil in a wok over moderate heat (just above middle flame, or medium on an electric setting). After 10 to 15 minutes test the oil by sticking something (a chopstick or a vegetable) in it. If the oil bubbles effusively it is ready.

Dip vegetables, seafood, or whatever in the batter 1 piece at a time and fry in the oil for 2 to 3 minutes until lightly golden. Don't fry more than 3 or 4 pieces at a time.

Place cooked vegetables on a paper towel to drain excess oil. Serve at once with dipping sauce.

# Vegetable Hummus

*The most famous of all Middle Eastern dishes, hummus means "chickpeas" in Arabic. This version is made with tahini* (hummus bi tahini), *but corn oil may be substituted for the tahini. Substitute roasted eggplant (sans skin) for the chickpeas and leave out the carrots to make baba ghanoush.*

2 cups cooked chickpeas (reserve some
   of the juice)
2 tablespoons tahini
2 cloves garlic, crushed
$1/4$ cup fresh lemon juice
Salt to taste
$1/2$ cup grated carrots
$1/2$ cup chopped parsley
I teaspoon paprika
Chopped parsley, as garnish
Paprika, as garnish

In a food processor, puree the chickpeas with the tahini, garlic, lemon juice, and salt. When the chickpea puree is almost smooth, add the rest of the ingredients and enough of the reserved chickpea juice to achieve dip consistency and process until well blended. (If you like chunky hummus, add another $1/2$ cup of chickpeas to the final mixture.)

Shape hummus into a mound on a serving plate or place in a bowl. Sprinkle with paprika and parsley and serve with crudités and pita wedges.

*I used to tell my vegan students that if they didn't learn to cook, hummus would be their fate. These days you can buy hummus—probably the most convenient protein-rich vegan food—just about anywhere. Add some pita bread and you've got an international fast-food fest. Not. I knew an animal rights activist who had a storehouse of empty hummus containers, I mean hun-dreds. The saying "Man does not live by bread alone" does not mean just add hummus and you're all set.*

# Nori Rolls

*These are easier to make than you would think, but it helps if you can get someone to show you how the first time. Ask the guy at the sushi bar or just watch very closely.*

4 sheets nori

2 cups sushi rice

1 $\frac{1}{2}$ tablespoons rice vinegar

1 tablespoon sweetener

1 teaspoon salt

1 carrot, cut in eighths lengthwise

4 long scallion greens

4 strips cucumber, peeled and cut
    lengthwise

2 tablespoons toasted sesame seeds

Soy sauce, for dipping

Wasabi, or wasabi powder mixed
    with a small amount of water

Rinse the rice and place in a 2-quart saucepan (or rice cooker) with 3 cups of water. Bring the rice to a boil, reduce heat to simmer, and cover the pot. Cook over low heat for about 20 minutes, until all water has evaporated.

Put the cooked rice in a large bowl to cool. Put the vinegar, sweetener, and salt in a small saucepan. Bring to a boil and turn off the heat. Add the vinegar mixture to the cooked rice and mix well.

Lay a sheet of nori down on a bamboo mat. Press one quarter of the rice evenly on top, leaving about 1 $\frac{1}{2}$ inches of nori space at the top and bottom.

Spread a small amount of wasabi across the middle of the rice. Place a strip each of cucumber, carrot, and scallion across the center of the rice, sprinkle with sesame seeds, and roll up. Slice the roll into 2-inch sections and serve with soy sauce to dip and wasabi to dash.

*Those sushi guys go to school for five years to learn their craft. They spend the first year just making rice and cleaning up. I love the obsession involved. Think of it, the freshest of the most perishable of foods, served over a seasoned rice that takes a year to perfect, and it looks like art! I'm not sure if it's heaven or time for more therapy.*

# Pad Chix Stix

*A variation on a Pad Thai theme. Try it with shrimp or scallops in place of chicken.*

3 tablespoons coconut milk
I tablespoon tomato paste
I tablespoon red wine vinegar
I tablespoon fish sauce
I tablespoon sweetener
I pound boneless chicken, cut into
    bite-sized chunks or strips
3 scallions, chopped
2 tablespoons finely chopped
    roasted peanuts
Bamboo skewers

In a large bowl, combine the coconut milk, tomato paste, red wine vinegar, fish sauce, and the sweetener as a marinade. Add the chicken. Marinate for 2 to 3 hours.

Place marinated chicken pieces on skewers and grill or broil for a few minutes on each side. Serve chicken skewers garnished with scallions and peanuts.

# Seviche

*The citrus juice cooks the fish. Really.*

$^1/_2$ pound shrimp, peeled and
    deveined
$^1/_2$ pound scallops
$^3/_4$ cup lime juice
2 tomatoes, diced
1 onion, diced fine
$^1/_2$ cup chopped cilantro leaves
1 teaspoon oregano
2 tablespoons olive oil, or less
1 jalapeño pepper, minced
Salt and pepper to taste

Combine all ingredients, mix well, and refrigerate. Let marinate for 6 to 24 hours and serve in parfait glasses or atop lettuce leaves.

*I hope there's a buffet in the hereafter. I love having all those choices. I've heard that my oral fixations and deep need for variety at the table may stem from a deficiency in other areas in my life. Whatever it is, it works for me. Everybody should be obsessed with at least one thing (aside from another person). It creates a kind of balance with the rest of the crazy world.*

# Oysters with Ponzu and Wasabi

*An indispensable part of a romantic dinner, these bivalves will light up your life. Ponzu sauce is a citrusy soy sauce that is delicious with seafood. You can find ponzu and wasabi at Oriental food stores and some natural food stores.*

3 to 6 oysters per person (don't get them too far in advance and ask your fish man to cut them and leave them in the shells for you—oyster cutting is dangerous for the uninitiated)
Green herbs, lemon wedges, red pepper strips, optional, as garnish
Wasabi powder
Ponzu sauce

Lay the oysters out on a platter. Garnish with green herbs, lemon wedges, and red pepper strips if desired.

Mix the wasabi powder with a small amount of water, a few drops at a time, to make a thick paste. Add a ball of wasabi paste to the plate of oysters. Put some ponzu sauce in a dipping cup with a serving spoon.

Put a dab of wasabi paste and a scant spoonful of ponzu on each oyster at the point of consumption. Love it.

*Tantalize your honey with a Valentine's Day feast. Try some oysters with ponzu sauce (a Japanese prepared sauce) and wasabi. I've always thought seafood was great for romance because fish seem so patient (waiting is a big part of romance from a male perspective). The main course is Salmon and Crab Rolls (p. 94) served with a Red Pepper Puree (p. 95). Serve some asparagus with the entree and finish off your Valentine fare with a heart-shaped strawberry-drenched almond cake (see p. 125). It's okay to be a little hokey on days like these. The expectation is bred in the bone, so go with it.*

# My Favorite Mussels

*Simple is best here. Let it be.*

*Mussels, fresh in their shells, rinsed, beards pulled*
*Freshly ground black pepper*
*Fine olive oil*

Clean the mussels and set aside. Heat an empty cast iron frying pan over high heat. When the pan is more than real hot, add the mussels (dry) and stir them around in the pan. When they open, after about 5 minutes, they're done. Give 'em a grind of black pepper and a drizzle of oil. Put the skillet on the table and dig in.

*Next time you feel annoyed at that waiter or waitress with the humongo pepper mill hovering over your shoulder in every restaurant you go to these days (except Oriental), remember the "spice story": Herbs and spices have essential oils within them that give them their flavor. At the moment the spice pods (or seeds, sticks, bark, or whatever) are broken up, their flavor is peak. So be nice to the pepper person.*

# Citrus Satay

*A delicious, easy-to-make, once-in-a-while kind of a dish.*

**For the marinade:**

2 cloves garlic
$1/4$ cup orange juice
1 tablespoon fish sauce
2 tablespoons coconut milk
1 teaspoon sweetener
$1/2$ teaspoon turmeric

**For something to marinate:**

1 pound boneless chicken cut into
    bite-sized pieces, or 1 pound whole
    shrimp or scallops

**For the dipping sauce:**

$1/2$ cup coconut milk
1 heaping teaspoon red Thai curry paste
1 to 1 $1/2$ tablespoons lime juice
2 teaspoons sweetener
2 teaspoons fish sauce
3 tablespoons peanut butter

Combine marinade ingredients and marinate the chicken for a few hours or overnight (if using seafood, don't marinate longer than 30 minutes).

In a separate bowl, whisk together all ingredients for the dipping sauce and set aside. (If you like your sauce more citrusy, sweet, or salty, add more juice, sweetener, or fish sauce to taste.)

Skewer the chicken or seafood and broil or grill to doneness. Serve skewers on a platter surrounding a bowl of dipping sauce.

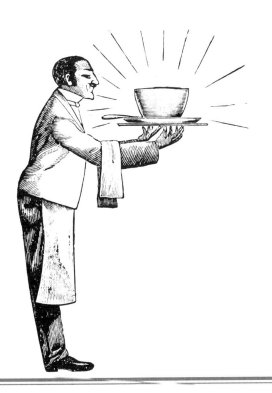

# SOUPS

# Miso-Ginger Udon

*The stock gives this traditional Japanese soup its rich, hearty flavor. Make vegetable stock by boiling mass quantities of vegetable scraps for an hour or more. (Use about 2 cups of veggie scraps for each quart of water.) All veggies are fair game for stock. I usually add a lot of fresh ginger to the stock for this soup as well as garlic, a bay leaf, and salt and pepper.*

2 quarts vegetable stock
4 tablespoons miso paste, or more
   to taste
1 onion, sliced
1 zucchini, sliced at an angle
2 carrots, sliced at an angle
$1/2$ bunch broccoli florets
$1/2$ pound cooked udon noodles
Chopped scallions, as garnish

Use a small amount of the stock to dilute the miso in a cup or small bowl and set aside. Place the stock, the sliced vegetables, and the broccoli florets in a large stock pot and bring to a low simmer. When the vegetables are tender add the diluted miso and the noodles and turn off the flame. Let sit for 5 to 10 minutes and then serve in individual bowls garnished with chopped scallions.

*I remember the first time I had a dish similar to this. It was at the old Open Sesame Restaurant—the haunt of the macro-faithfuls—in Brookline, Massachusetts. Followers of Mr. Kushi and Mac wanna-bes alike groovin' together over bancha tea and a blissful number of sanctioned desserts. It was a scene that I am grateful to have passed through and passed on. It was sort of a cult, but cults are fun for a while. You get to hang out with like-minded individuals and eat a lot. I wonder, where have all the macros gone and what are they eating these days?*

# Middle Eastern Black-eyed Pea Soup

*Black-eyed peas are one of the "beans" (actually a legume) I like to cook because they don't require overnight soaking. The combination of flavors here is outstanding.*

2 tablespoons olive oil

1 onion, chopped

8 ounces black-eyed peas

1 jalapeño pepper, minced (use
    more if you like it hot)

3 or 4 cloves of garlic, minced

1 tablespoon cumin

1 teaspoon turmeric

5 cups stock or water

Salt and pepper to taste

1 large tomato, chopped

$^1/_2$ cup fresh cilantro leaves, chopped

$^1/_4$ cup lemon juice, or more to taste

Plain yogurt, optional

Heat the oil in a large stock pot. Add the onion and sauté until slightly browned.

Add the black-eyed peas, the minced jalapeño, and the garlic and sauté for another minute or so. Add the cumin and turmeric and sauté 1 additional minute.

Add the stock and bring the pot to a boil. Add salt and pepper, reduce the heat to a strong simmer, and cook until the peas are tender, about 45 minutes.

Add the tomato and the cilantro, turn off the flame, stir, and let sit for 10 to 15 minutes. Add the lemon juice and serve, garnished with a dollop of plain yogurt if desired.

# Squash Soup

*Have fun with squash. You can make this soup with any type of winter squash, yams, sweet potatoes, or a combination.*

3 cups winter squash, peeled and
   cut into 2-inch cubes
6 cups stock or 6 cups water and
   squash water (the water squash
   was boiled in)
1 tablespoon vegetable oil, or more
2 large onions, sliced
Salt and pepper to taste
Spices to taste, choose from:
   Pumpkin pie spice
   Cinnamon
   Curry powder
   Fresh ginger
   Five-spice powder (my favorite)
Plain yogurt, optional as garnish

Boil the squash in stock or water until soft.

Heat the oil in a sauté pan and fry the sliced onion until browned.

Strain the squash and puree with the onion and $1/4$ to $1/2$ cup of the squash water in a food processor and add salt and pepper to taste. While processing, add more of the boiling liquid or stock to achieve desired (it's up to you) consistency and any of the optional spices to taste.

Serve with a dollop of yogurt, or mix the yogurt into the soup for a creamier version.

# Florentine White Bean Soup

*Beans and greens = big fun. This soup is especially good made with chicken stock.*

6 cups stock, chicken or veg
2 cups navy beans, cooked
1 zucchini, cut into half-moons
1 onion, sliced
1 carrot, cut into matchsticks
$1/2$ teaspoon each (or more)
   marjoram, basil, and oregano
Salt and pepper to taste
$1/2$ pound spinach, washed and
   chopped
$1/2$ pound spinach noodles, cooked
Lemon juice

Combine the stock, beans, zucchini, onion, carrot, spices, and salt and pepper in a large soup pot and bring to a gentle simmer over medium heat. When the vegetables are tender add the spinach and the noodles and turn off the heat. Let sit for a few minutes and serve hot with a squeeze of fresh lemon juice.

# Sunset Soup

*A hearty favorite. The red lentils and the flesh of the yellow-orange squash turn sunset orange. Add a beet for more red.*

1 tablespoon or more olive oil
1 onion, chopped
1 cup red lentils
1 medium butternut squash (or
    other sweet winter), peeled and
    cut into 1-inch cubes
1 tablespoon cumin powder
1 1/2 teaspoons coriander
6 cups stock or water
2 bay leaves
Salt to taste
Plain yogurt, optional garnish

Heat the oil in a heavy-bottomed stock pot and fry the onion until lightly browned. Add the lentils and the squash and continue to fry while stirring for a few minutes.

Add the cumin and coriander and sauté 1 minute longer.

Add the stock, bay leaves, and salt and bring the pot to a boil. Reduce the heat to a simmer and cook until the lentils are tender, about 50 minutes. Check for seasoning, adjust to taste, and serve, garnished with a dollop of plain yogurt if desired.

 **TIP**

*Spices come from the seed of the plant and herbs come from the leaf. In general, the seeds have a heartier texture and can be sautéed directly in oil; the leaves are more delicate and should be added to other ingredients later in the cooking process.*

# Seafood Gumbo

*This one is much "more better" tomorrow.*

1 pound shrimp, peeled and
    deveined (save the shells)
8 cups water
2 tablespoons vegetable oil
4 tablespoons white flour
1 small onion, chopped
4 cloves garlic, chopped
1 green bell pepper, chopped
2 stalks celery, chopped
1 cup tomato sauce
1 10-ounce package frozen sliced okra
1 teaspoon thyme
3 bay leaves
Salt and pepper to taste
$1/2$ pound crabmeat
$1/2$ cup chopped parsley, as garnish
Cooked white rice,
    as accompaniment

Preheat oven to 400°F.

Roast the shrimp shells on a cookie sheet in preheated oven until lightly browned and crispy, about 15 minutes. Place the water in a large soup pot and boil the roasted shells for about 45 minutes to make a stock. Strain the stock, discard the shells, and set the shrimp stock aside.

In a large pot with a heavy bottom, heat the oil, add the flour, and sauté over medium-low heat, stirring and frying until the flour gets a bit more than lightly browned and sweet and nutty smellin'. Add the onion, garlic, pepper, and celery and continue to sauté until the onion becomes translucent. Add the tomato sauce, okra, herbs, and salt and pepper and continue stirring and frying for a few minutes. Pour in the shrimp stock, the shrimp, and the crabmeat and simmer over low heat for about 30 minutes.

Serve in individual bowls with a scoop of white rice, garnished with chopped parsley.

*Bay leaves are the dried leaves of the laurel. The bay leaf is the most noble herb. The ancient Greeks crowned their heroes with laurel. The expression "resting on one's laurels" comes from the tradition of crowning Greek and Roman victors with crowns of laurel—after their great feats they could rest until the next challenge. Here's a recipe for success: stuff a mattress full of bay leaves. Rest.*

# Thai Chicken-Coconut Soup

*Here's a rich one. This is my favorite Thai soup and it's easy to make.*

3 cups chicken broth
Zest of 1 lemon
3 thin slices fresh ginger (or galingale)
3 tablespoons Thai fish sauce
3 tablespoons lime juice (or more to taste)
2 tablespoons sweetener
1 can unsweetened coconut milk
$3/4$ pound boneless chicken, cut into thin strips
1 jalapeño pepper, seeded and chopped fine
3 tablespoons cilantro leaves, shredded, as garnish

Combine all ingredients except the cilantro in a soup pot and simmer until the chicken is cooked. Garnish with cilantro and serve hot.

# Gazpacho

*Each region of Spain has its own version of this famous dish. Gazpacho is not really a soup but a sip.*

8 large, ripe tomatoes (or 2 large
   cans of imported), diced
1 cucumber, peeled and diced
1 green bell pepper, diced
3 cloves garlic, chopped
3 teaspoons olive oil
3 tablespoons white wine or sherry
   wine vinegar
3 tablespoons fresh lemon juice
1 teaspoon salt
Freshly ground black pepper
Tabasco sauce to taste, optional
$1/_2$ cup water
Sliced cucumber, as garnish
Fresh sprigs of parsley, as garnish
Croutons, as garnish

Puree all ingredients in a food processor. Serve garnished with a slice of cucumber, a sprig of parsley, and a sprinkle of croutons.

*Gazpacho is a good example of regional cuisine, meaning dishes that are created from whatever foodstuffs are available (seasonally speaking) particular to that part of the world. For example, coq au vin (chicken in wine) is a dish from the French countryside making use of locally raised chicken, local wines, and home-grown carrots, mushrooms, onions, and garlic. Regional cuisine is very popular in this country because we are attracted to the idea of its authenticity (even if it's presented in a tacky manner). Look at a map the next time you eat a regional dish and imagine yourself in that locale. Far out!*

# Black Bean Soup

*Cuban delight.*

3 cups dry black beans
3 quarts water
Salt
1 bay leaf
1 tablespoon cumin
1 tablespoon oregano
5 cloves garlic, minced
1 tablespoon soy sauce
1 tablespoon olive oil (or more)
1 large onion, chopped
1 large green bell pepper, chopped
1 tablespoon vinegar
Cooked white rice, as garnish
Chopped red onion, as garnish
Olive oil, optional

Soak the beans in water overnight.

Drain the soaking water, rinse the beans and place them in a soup pot with the 3 quarts of water, the salt, and the bay leaf, and bring to a boil. After 1 hour add the cumin, oregano, garlic, and soy sauce. Reduce the heat to a simmer and continue to cook the beans until soft and very tender, about 30 minutes. Meanwhile, heat the oil in a frying pan and sauté the onion and pepper until soft and browned. Add the sautéed pepper and onion and the vinegar to the beans, turn off the heat, and let soup sit to blend flavors before serving. Serve soup in individual bowls with a scoop of white rice and some chopped raw red onion. Top with olive oil and more vinegar if desired.

# Chinatown Chicken Noodle Soup

*Quick to cook and long on flavor.*

1 pound boneless chicken thighs
1 tablespoon dark sesame oil or other
    vegetable oil
3 tablespoons minced ginger
3 cloves garlic, minced
$^1/_4$ cup cream sherry
3 tablespoons or less soy sauce
2 teaspoons dry sweetener
6 cups chicken stock (or part stock,
    part water, or all water if you
    must)
4 ounces fresh Chinese noodles (the
    thin ones)
1 large portabello mushroom (or 4
    ounces other mushrooms), thinly
    sliced
Scallion greens, chopped

Cut each chicken thigh into 6 chunks. Heat the oil in a large saucepan and add the chicken and the ginger. Stir and fry (searing but not letting it stick) until the chicken is browned a bit.

Add the garlic and cook 30 seconds longer. Add the sherry, soy sauce, and dry sweetener and bring to a boil to form a sauce base. Add the stock and bring to a boil again.

Add the noodles and turn the heat down to a medium simmer. Cook until the noodles are al dente, about 5 minutes, add the mushroom slices, and turn off the heat. Serve garnished with chopped scallion.

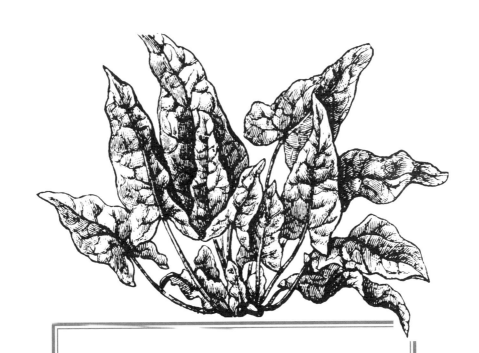

# SALADS

# Warm Citrus Shrimp Vinaigrette

*Try a warm dressing for a change of pace. Fresh herbs and citrus are a taste explosion. Bay scallops (the small ones) work well in this dish too.*

Juice of 1 orange and 1 teaspoon
   zest
Juice of 1 lemon and $1/2$ teaspoon
   zest
2 tablespoons olive oil
1 tablespoon chopped fresh sage
   leaf (or 1 teaspoon dry sage)
1 teaspoon fresh coriander root,
   minced fine (or $1/2$ teaspoon dry
   coriander)
1 ripe tomato, diced
2 scallions, chopped
Salt and pepper to taste
1 pound medium shrimp, peeled
   and deveined
Salad greens for 4

Combine the citrus juices and zest with the olive oil, herbs, diced tomato, scallions, and salt and pepper in a saucepan and bring almost to a boil. Add the shrimp, stir, and turn off the heat. Let sit until the shrimp are firm and fully cooked, about 5 minutes. Divide the salad greens onto separate plates and dress with shrimp and sauce.

# Marinated Tomato Salad

*Simple and pretty, a lovely side dish.*

4 large ripe, red tomatoes, sliced fairly
  thin
2 tablespoons white wine vinegar
2 tablespoons or less olive oil
$1/2$ teaspoon dry marjoram (or 2
  teaspoons fresh)
$1/2$ teaspoon dry tarragon (or 2
  teaspoons fresh)
2 scallions, chopped
2 tablespoons chopped fresh Italian (flat)
  parsley
Salt and pepper to taste

Place the tomato slices on a glass plate in an attractive manner.

Combine all other ingredients in a bottle to shake, or in a bowl to stir, and pour over the tomatoes. Cover and chill for 1 to 2 hours before serving.

# TIP

*If a recipe calls for fresh herbs and you don't have any, use the about $1/3$ to $1/2$ amount of dry. Fresh herbs are more flavorful. Dry are much more dense.*

# Oriental Broccoli Salad

*A great vegetable dish to serve with Oriental foods. The taste of soy sauce and ginger works well with Japanese or Chinese dishes. Buy the dark sesame oil for this dish and use it again for Five-Spice Turkey Tenders (p. 121). You can make a great Oriental-style dressing too, using half dark sesame oil and half lemon juice.*

1 bunch broccoli, cut into thin, long-stemmed florets

2 tablespoons soy sauce

2 tablespoons rice vinegar

1 teaspoon sweetener

1 clove garlic, minced fine

1 tablespoon fresh ginger, grated or minced fine

1 tablespoon dark sesame oil (plus a dash of hot oil for more spice if desired)

Black pepper to taste

1 tablespoon sesame seeds, dry-toasted in a fry pan

Steam the broccoli until al dente.

Combine all other ingredients (except sesame seeds), add the broccoli, and marinate in the fridge for at least 30 minutes. (For a warm dish, drizzle combined ingredients over just-steamed broccoli and serve immediately.) Garnish, warm or cold, with sesame seeds before serving.

# Eggplant Salad

*Serve with toasted bread or as a garnish for grilled chicken or fish. A tasty veggie side dish. The sherry wine vinegar gives the salad a distinctive and rich Spanish flavor. Buy it for this dish and use it in Gazpacho (p. 23). Serve Gazpacho and Paella (p. 83) with this Eggplant Salad for a Spanish food fest.*

1 large eggplant
1 tablespoon olive oil
1 small onion, chopped
1 red bell pepper, chopped
2 small tomatoes, chopped
1 teaspoon sweetener
1 tablespoon sherry wine vinegar
1 tablespoon capers
Salt and pepper to taste

Preheat oven to 400°F.

Poke a few holes in the eggplant and roast it in the preheated oven until soft, about 45 minutes. Heat the olive oil in a frying pan, add the onion and the pepper, and sauté until they begin to brown.

Cut the roasted eggplant into bite-sized cubes and add it to the onion and peppers along with the chopped tomatoes. Continue to sauté for 2 to 3 minutes. Add all the other ingredients, turn off the heat, and let sit for at least 30 minutes before serving.

# Shrimp Salad Rémoulade

*Try this dish with crab instead of shrimp for variety. Omit the horseradish for a milder version.*

1 tablespoon prepared mustard
1 tablespoon lemon juice
1 teaspoon paprika
2 cloves garlic
1 tablespoon prepared horseradish
3 tablespoons olive oil
1 pound shrimp, peeled and cooked
1 bell pepper, chopped fine
3 stalks celery, chopped fine
1 bunch scallions, chopped
Lettuce leaves
Chopped parsley, as garnish

Combine the mustard, lemon, paprika, garlic, and horseradish in a large bowl. Slowly drizzle in the oil and whisk to thicken. Add the shrimp, pepper, celery, and scallions to the dressing and toss.

Spoon the shrimp salad on lettuce leaves for individual servings and garnish with chopped parsley.

*The word* gourmet *comes from the French tax collection services of the Middle Ages. The king was entitled to ten percent of a citizen's crops. The tax collector took the best ten percent. Gourmet came to mean the person (tax collector) who selected the cream of the crop. No wonder the word sounds so elitist. It is, but in a good way. It means someone who cares to select the best of what is currently available. Go into the grocery store with an elitist attitude. Select only the best merchandise. If everyone did this, the stores would raise their standards. All stores would be gourmet.*

# Sweet Potato Salad

*Everybody loves this—a great "What are you bringing?" for Thanksgiving.*

3 large sweet potatoes or yams, cut
   into steak-fry-sized strips
2 tablespoons olive oil
Salt and pepper to taste
1 bunch scallions (greens only),
   chopped
1 $^1/_2$ tablespoons apple cider vinegar

Preheat the oven to 425°F.

Put the potatoes in a large baking dish. Drizzle with olive oil and sprinkle with salt and pepper. Bake in preheated oven until lightly browned and slightly soft, about 40 minutes. Combine the cooked potatoes with the vinegar and scallions in a serving dish. Serve hot, cold, or at room temperature.

# Thai Cucumber Salad

*This salad has a cooling effect that goes well with spicy foods. Try it with Green Curry Chicken (p. 110).*

1 large cucumber, peeled, scored,
   and sliced
Juice of 1 lime
1 teaspoon sweetener
1 tablespoon fish sauce
1 carrot, cut into thin matchsticks
$^1/_2$ red onion, sliced into very thin
   half-moons
2 plum tomatoes, sliced thin
2 tablespoons cilantro leaves,
   chopped
Cilantro sprigs, as garnish
Crushed roasted peanuts, as garnish

Combine all ingredients except cilantro and peanuts in a salad bowl and toss gently. Serve garnished with whole sprigs of cilantro and crushed peanuts.

# Middle Eastern Date and Orange Salad

*A refreshing change of pace. Almost a dessert salad.*

2 tablespoons lemon juice
3 tablespoons orange juice
   concentrate
2 tablespoons olive oil
$1/2$ teaspoon cinnamon
Pinch of salt
1 large heart of romaine lettuce
   (mostly the white part), shredded
3 navel oranges, sectioned, sections
   cut in half
$1 1/2$ cups chopped dates (chop your own)
$1/2$ cup toasted almond slivers, as garnish

Mix the lemon juice, orange juice concentrate, olive oil, cinnamon, and salt to make a dressing. In a large bowl, combine the lettuce and fruits and toss with the dressing. Garnish with toasted almonds.

# Fattoush

*A Lebanese summer vegetable and bread salad. It's a substantial and refreshing side dish because it combines starch (the bread) and fresh summer veggies. Serve it at your next BBQ.*

1 cup ripe diced tomato
1 cup peeled and diced cucumber
$1/2$ cup finely diced red onion
2 tablespoons chopped fresh mint
2 tablespoons chopped fresh
    parsley
1 large pita bread, toasted and cut
    into 1-inch squares
2 tablespoons olive oil
3 tablespoons lemon juice
2 teaspoons balsamic vinegar
$1/2$ teaspoon orange zest
Salt and pepper to taste
Sprigs of mint, as garnish

In a large salad bowl, mix together the tomato, cucumber, onion, mint, parsley, and toasted bread squares. Combine all other ingredients to make a dressing and toss together. Garnish with whole sprigs of mint.

# TIP

*Don't buy a set of knives, even if they're on sale—nothing's a bargain if you don't need it. Instead, spend your money on a good chef's knife (the one you'll use all the time). Sets tend to only gather dust and clutter up the kitchen.*

# Carrot Salad with Mint

*A refreshing way to eat healthy carrots on a hot summer day. Add a pinch of cinnamon for some Middle Eastern flair.*

2 tablespoons lemon juice
1 tablespoon red wine vinegar
2 tablespoons choppped fresh mint
   sprigs
2 tablespoons olive oil
Salt
Pinch of sweetener
2 cups carrot matchsticks (or large-
   grated or food-processed)
Mint sprigs, as garnish

Combine liquid ingredients with seasonings, dress carrots, and refrigerate for 1 hour. Serve chilled, garnished with mint sprigs.

## TIP

*The best way to keep fresh herbs is alive in their own little pots. You can pick them as needed. They cost about the same this way as those packets you buy at the grocery store. If you have leftover fresh herbs, use them to flavor olive oil (immerse herbs in oil for 24 hours) for dipping breads, sautéing, and marinating.*

# Thai Pineapple-Chicken Salad

*More fun with pineapple. Serve this with shredded lettuce as a salad or roll portions of it up inside whole lettuce leaves for appetizers. You'll be glad you did. I love it.*

1 tablespoon peanut oil
1 onion, finely chopped
1 pound boneless chicken thighs,
  cut into small bite-sized pieces
2 or 3 cloves garlic, minced
1 jalapeño pepper, seeded and
  chopped fine
1 can crushed pineapple
2 tablespoons Thai fish sauce
1 head Bibb lettuce, shredded or broken
  into whole leaves
$1/2$ cup roasted peanuts, crushed
$1/4$ cup chopped cilantro leaves

Heat the oil in a frying pan. Add the onion and sauté for a few minutes. Add the chicken, the garlic, and the jalapeño pepper and continue to fry, stirring until lightly browned, 5 to 7 minutes.

Add the the can of pineapple (with juice) and the fish sauce to the pan and cook for a few more minutes. To serve as a salad, spoon the chick-mix (warm or cooled) over shredded lettuce or wrap a bit in a single whole lettuce leaf to serve as an appetizer, as many as you like. Either way, serve garnished with crushed peanuts and cilantro.

# TIP

*You can use less oil than a recipe calls for when stir-frying. If the pan gets dry, add 1 tablespoon at a time of liquid (soy sauce, stock, balsamic vinegar, water, wine, or whatever) and continue stirring and frying. Don't add too much liquid—it will reduce the temperature in the pan and you'll end up with a soggy simmer.*

# Bitter Greens Salad with Orange-Sesame Dressing

*Bitter is better. Try this at the end of dinner as a digestif.*

**For salad:**

3 cups greens, any combination,
   choose from:
      Endive
      Escarole
      Radicchio
      Dandelion greens

**For dressing:**

Juice of 1 orange
1 teaspoon rice vinegar
2 tablespoons dark sesame oil
1 tablespoon soy sauce
$1/2$ teaspoon lemon zest
Freshly ground pepper to taste
1 tablespoon toasted sesame seeds

Combine all ingredients for dressing, drizzle over greens, toss, and serve.

# Sherry Shallot Chicken Salad

*This dish is pure Madison Avenue bistro food, à la française. Serve it warm for maximum taste effect. Simple and elegant.*

3 tablespoons olive oil

3 tablespoons sherry wine vinegar

1 teaspoon Dijon-style mustard

2 shallots, chopped

Salt and pepper to taste

1 pound boneless chicken, cut into
    pinkie-sized strips

$1/4$ pound mixed salad greens or
    mesclun mix

$1/2$ cup carrot matchsticks

1 cup herb croutons (see below)

Preheat oven to 400°F.

In a small bowl, combine the oil, vinegar, mustard, chopped shallots, and salt and pepper to taste.

Place the chicken strips in a baking dish in a single layer and pour the oil-vinegar mix over it. Add a few tablespoons of water to the dish and bake in preheated oven for 12 to 15 minutes. Place the salad greens, the carrots, and the croutons in a large salad bowl and toss.

When the chicken is cooked, dress the salad with the hot juices from the baking dish and arrange the chicken on top of the dressed greens in an attractive manner.

**To make herb croutons:** Cut herbed bread into 1-inch cubes, place on a baking tray, drizzle with olive oil, and toast until lightly browned. If herbed bread is not available, cube a baguette, drizzle with olive oil, sprinkle with a little thyme, dill, and sage, and toast until browned.

# Mesclun Salad with Raspberry Vinaigrette and Shrimp Hearts

*This simple salad of sparkling, fresh ingredients will be sure to win the heart of your intended.*

24 large shrimp, peeled and
    deveined
2 tablespoons rasyberry wine vinegar
Squeeze of lemon juice
Pinch of sweetener
Pinch of fresh ground pepper
4 tablespoons extra-virgin olive oil
$^1/_2$ pound mesclun greens or other
    mixed salad greens such as
    arugula, radicchio, romaine, Bibb,
    red leaf
1 handful fresh or frozen raspberrries
Edible flowers, optional, as garnish

Steam the shrimp for 2 to 3 minutes and set aside.

Place a handful of salad greens on individual plates. To arrange the shrimp as hearts, take 2 shrimp and place them head to head and tail to tail. Place 3 shrimp hearts, or pairs, around each salad.

In a small bowl, combine the vinegar, lemon juice, sweetener, and pepper and whisk in the oil. Add the berries to the dressing and stir. Dress and serve individual salads garnished with edible flowers if available.

*"I'm a freelance, part-time, bonafide food stylist."*
*"Food stylist," you say, how interesting. "What the hell is that?"*
*"Well," I explain, "I shellac French fries, spray turkeys with food coloring, and dish detergent, Crazy-Glue the parts back on lobsters (don't ask), use Elmer's glue for milk, you know, whatever I have to do to make it look good on TV. On cooking shows, I'm the guy behind the guy, behind the guy. Sometimes I make a hundred of whatever they're selling and they pick one. I play with food and I'm probably the person you're going to call when you want to do something different with your turkey this year."*
*"Oh really."*

# Roasted Garlic Dressing

*When preparing this dressing, roast extra garlic bulbs to use as a spread for breadsticks. Just dip in and eat a hunk of garlic: you'll be glad you did. Roasting garlic makes it sweet and milder than the raw stuff. You can use it in place of raw garlic in any recipe.*

1 whole bulb of garlic (preferably
   with large cloves)
$1/2$ cup olive oil
Salt and pepper to taste
2 tablespoons balsamic vinegar

Preheat oven to 350°F.

Cut the garlic bulb in half across the middle. Rub it inside and out with 1 teaspoon of the oil and sprinkle lightly with salt. Place the garlic halves back together, wrap the bulb in tin foil, and bake in preheated oven for 1 hour.

In a small bowl, blend 3 to 5 roasted garlic cloves with the vinegar. Whisk in the remaining olive oil and add salt and pepper to taste.

# Asparagus Vinaigrette

*A tangy international side dish. Add it to your next paella feast.*

2 tablespoons olive oil
2 tablespoons red wine vinegar
1 teaspoon Dijon mustard
2 tablespoons roasted almonds
1 pound fresh asparagus, ends
  trimmed
Salt and pepper to taste

In a small bowl, whisk together the oil, vinegar, mustard, and salt and pepper and set aside.

Steam or blanch the asparagus until tender but not limp. Rinse under cold water to cool (or serve hot). Toss the asparagus with the dressing, garnish with crushed almonds, and serve.

# Ensalada Tri Colore

*The idea here is to display the colors of the Italian flag—*rosso, bianco, e verde.

*Use equal portions or in amounts*
*preferred:*
*Radicchio*
*Arugula*
*Endive*
*Extra-virgin olive oil*
*Balsamic vinegar*

Chop the vegetables and arrange them by color on a large platter. Dress with equal amounts of oil and vinegar.

## TIP

*Pricey extra-virgin olive oil should be used as a condiment. If you heat the oil above 140°F, as you would for most types of cooking, it will lose the subtle qualities that it's most valued for. Use pure olive oil or an inexpensive extra-virgin oil for cooking.*

# Tomatillo Salad

*Make use of the exotic. A great Mexi side dish.*

10 fresh tomatillos, sliced
1 large ripe red tomato, halved and sliced
1 cucumber, sliced
1 bunch scallions, chopped
2 tablespoons olive oil
3 tablespoons red wine vinegar
1 clove garlic, minced
Salt and pepper to taste
Fresh sage leaves for garnish

Combine vegetables in a salad bowl. In a separate, small bowl, whisk the oil into the vinegar, add the garlic, and season with salt and pepper. Dress vegetables, toss lightly to coat, and serve garnished with fresh sage.

# Fresh Spinach with Lemon-Sesame Sauce

*Imagine Popeye Japanese.*

1 pound fresh spinach, washed,
    stems removed, coarsely chopped
2 tablespoons sesame tahini
3 tablespoons freshly squeezed lemon
    juice
1 tablespoon soy sauce
Sesame seeds
Scallion greens, sliced thin

Lightly grease 2 custard cups.

Blanch the spinach in boiling water for a few seconds (keep it green). Rinse under cold water, pat dry, and stuff into the greased custard cups. Refrigerate for at least 1 hour.

Combine the tahini, lemon juice, and soy sauce in a bowl and blend well. Unmold the spinach onto 2 small plates, dress with lemon-tahini sauce, and garnish with sesame seeds and scallions.

# Orange-Ginger Spinach Salad with Scallops

*This marinade works very well with most types of seafood. You'll want to try it again—the mustard grows on you.*

**For the marinade:**

$3/4$ cup fresh orange juice
2 teaspoons Dijon mustard
2 tablespoons olive oil
1 tablespoon fresh ginger, minced
Salt and pepper to taste

**For the salad:**

1 pound sea scallops
8 ounces fresh spinach leaves,
    washed and chopped
1 large carrot, cut into matchsticks
2 scallions, chopped
Croutons, optional

In a glass bowl or baking dish, combine the marinade ingredients. Add the scallops to the marinade, toss lightly to coat, and marinate for 30 minutes.

Combine the spinach, carrot, scallions, and croutons in a salad bowl and toss. Arrange on individual salad plates if desired.

Broil the marinated scallops for 6 to 10 minutes (depending on size of scallops). Pour the broiled scallops and pan juices over the salad ingredients and serve warm.

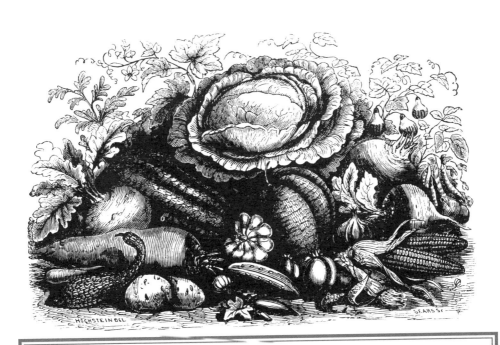

# VEGETABLES

# Collard Greens with Mustard Vinaigrette

*A fancy way to serve the underrated collard. Another Thanksgiving bring-along.*

12 ounces collard greens, confetti
  cut, stems removed
1 tablespoon balsamic vinegar
1 teaspoon Dijon mustard
2 teaspoons sweetener
Salt and pepper to taste
1 tablespoon olive oil
2 scallion greens, chopped
1/4 cup pecans, toasted and chopped

Steam the collards until tender, about 5 to 7 minutes.

Meanwhile, mix the vinegar with the mustard, sweetener, and salt and pepper and whisk in the oil to make a dressing.

Toss the steamed greens with the dressing, garnish with chopped scallions and pecans, and serve hot.

*Organic foods are more expensive than conventionally grown foods because they're more labor-intensive to produce. I know that when you look at packages of a conventionally produced food product, it seems like you get more stuff, but it's just stuff. The chemicals used in conventional-food production methods control the process to require less hands-on attention. Organic foods require a lot more care. When you buy organic foods, you're casting a vote for more caring in the marketplace.*

# String Beans with Fresh Mint

*Good stuff from the garden. A tasty Yankee side dish.*

*1 pound fresh string beans, left long, ends cut, and cleaned*

*2 tablespoons olive oil*

*2 tablespoons red wine vinegar*

*1 clove garlic, minced*

*Salt and pepper to taste*

*2 tablespoons chopped mint leaves*

Boil the beans in salted water for about 5 minutes until tender but still crisp (steaming is okay too).

In a small bowl, combine the oil, vinegar, and minced garlic and add salt and pepper to taste.

Dress the still-hot beans with the oil and vinegar mix, add the chopped mint leaves, and toss. Serve hot as a side dish or chill and serve as a salad.

# Middle Eastern Veggie Stew

*This stew can be made with all types of vegetables. Try it with okra, celery, green beans, or a combination. To serve as a main course, add a pound of boneless chicken thighs cut into larger-than-bite-sized chunks.*

1 teaspoon olive oil
1 large onion, diced large
1 large carrot, cut into $^1/_2$-inch
   rounds
1 branch broccoli, separated into
   large florets
1 large portabello mushroom, cut in
   half and thickly sliced
1 crumbled bay leaf
Salt and pepper to taste
1 teaspoon cinnamon
1 28-ounce can peeled tomatoes
   with their juice

In a wok or large sauté pan, heat the oil and fry the onion over medium heat until it begins to brown. Add the other vegetables (and the chicken if desired) and continue to fry, stirring, for a few minutes. (If the pan gets dry, add a little liquid—water or tomato juice—1 tablespoon at a time.) Add the salt and pepper, the crumbled bay leaf, cinnamon, and tomatoes with their juice to the pan and bring to a low boil. Turn the heat down to low and simmer the vegetables (and chicken) until tender. *Fini.*

# TIP

*If someone in your house wants to eat a low-fat vegetarian meal and you don't, here's the solution: Make the low-fat veggie meal for two and cook some marinated chicken (or whatever) on the side. Serve the veggies to the veggie (add some canned beans for protein if desired) and pour the chicken with pan juices over yours.*

# Corn with Chili and Lime

*Roast the corn in the oven or grill it on the … you know.*

*Fresh ears of corn, husk left on*
*Limes, quartered*
*Chili powder*

Preheat the oven to 550°F or light up the grill. Place the corn, still in its husk, on the oven rack or grill grate. When grilling, turn the corn often to avoid burning. Cook the corn until tender but not soft, about 20 minutes.

To serve, pull down the husk (you can use it as a handle), squirt with lime juice, and dust with chili powder.

# Stir-Fried Watercress

*Don't cook it too long. Keep it mean and green.*

1 tablespoon or less peanut or
  sesame oil
1 2-inch piece fresh ginger root, cut
  into small chunks
2 cloves garlic, chopped
2 bunches watercress, washed well
  with thick stems removed
1 tablespoon soy sauce
Pinch of black or white pepper

Heat the oil over high heat in a wok or frying pan large enough to contain the watercress. Add the ginger and fry for 1 minute. Add the garlic and fry for 30 seconds. Add the watercress and stir and fry for about 1 more minute. Add the soy sauce and pepper and serve immediately.

# TIP

*Buy plenty of spoons and stir-fry tools made of wood. They're cheap and won't scratch up a pan. Leave them near the stove for a quick grab in the heat of the moment.*

# Veggie Ribbons with Yogurt Sauce

*A novel side dish with an uplifting flavor.*

1 large zucchini
2 large carrots
Juice of 1 lemon
1 teaspoon dry thyme (or 1
    tablespoon fresh leaves)
Salt and pepper to taste
1 cup non-fat plain yogurt

Using a good-quality peeler, peel the zucchini and the carrots into long thin strips, making veggie ribbons.

In a small bowl or straight in the yogurt container, add the lemon juice and seasonings to the cup of yogurt and stir with a fork until smooth (add a little water if it seems too thick).

Steam the veggie ribbons to desired doneness.

Microwave the yogurt sauce for 1 minute, pour over the ribbons, and serve.

# Roasted Eggplant with Garlic

*Have fun with your eggplant and make a friend of garlic. This is the main course in vegan heaven.*

2 eggplants, left whole
8 cloves garlic, quartered lengthwise
1 bunch fresh thyme
Salt and pepper to taste
Olive oil
Lemon juice

Preheat oven to 400°F.

In each eggplant, make 16 slits large enough to insert a piece of garlic and a small herb sprig. Plant a piece of garlic and a sprig of thyme into each slit and bake the eggplants in the preheated oven for 35 to 45 minutes.

Quarter each eggplant lengthwise and serve hot—drizzled with olive oil, dashed with salt and pepper, and spritzed with lemon juice.

# Sardinian Vegetable Sauté

*Olive oil is the key here. Use a good one.*

1 head cauliflower, cut into small florets
1 head broccoli, cut into small florets
2 carrots, sliced
$^1/_2$ cup olive oil (or less if you gotta)
4 cloves garlic, minced
1 tablespoon anchovy paste
Salt and pepper to taste
2 tablespoons lemon juice
2 teaspoons lemon zest
$^1/_2$ cup pine nuts, toasted

Blanch the vegetables in boiling water until tender, about 2 minutes.

Gently heat the oil in a large sauté pan or wok, add the garlic and anchovy paste, and cook for 1 minute (don't let the garlic get dark). Add the vegetables to the pan and fry, stirring, for a few minutes. Add the salt and pepper and turn off the heat.

Toss the vegetables with the lemon juice and lemon zest, garnish with pine nuts, and serve.

*We used to laugh at my grandmother because she could never throw away leftover food. Lost among the ginger ale and meat loaf, there always seemed to be a bowl in her refrigerator with three peas in it. My grandparents on both sides were grocers and had a great respect for food. Food was the source of life and the essence of all that is hopeful and good. I didn't realize it at the time, but when grandma had a few generations of family around the dining room table, she was living her dream. I can see her now, smiling beatifically from the chair nearest the kitchen, the table before her laden with the foods that nourished the soul of the family. And it was good.*

# Oven-"Fried" Okra

*Sorta like Shake'n Bake but better. This is an alternative to frying that really works. "And I helped."*

1 cup bread crumbs
Salt and pepper to taste
2 eggs, beaten (or 3 egg whites)
Tabasco sauce to taste
1 pound fresh okra pods

Preheat oven to 475°F.

Put the bread crumbs in a large bowl and add salt and pepper to taste.

In a separate bowl, stir the Tabasco into the beaten egg. Dunk a few okra pods at a time in the egg then toss lightly to coat in the crumbs. Place crumbed okra on a greased cookie sheet and bake in preheated oven for about 10 minutes or until brown and crispy.

# Orange-Flavored Spinach with Pine Nuts

*A nice twist on spinach. If you can't find orange blossom water, use a half teaspoon of orange zest and a dash of orange juice.*

1 tablespoon or more olive oil
1 pound fresh spinach, washed and
    chopped medium
1 tablespoon orange blossom water
Salt and pepper to taste
Dash nutmeg
$1/4$ cup pine nuts, toasted and chopped
    coarse

Heat the olive oil in a large frying pan. Add the spinach to the oil and sauté until it wilts but retains a bright green color. Add the orange blossom water to the pan and toss.

Salt and pepper to taste, dash with nutmeg, garnish with pine nuts, and serve.

## TIP

*In a stir-fry situation, wait until the pan and the oil are heated through before adding any of the other ingredients—you want to hear that sizzle. That means the food is getting pan-seared and not just soaking up oil.*

# Marjoram Mushrooms

*A great way to enjoy mushrooms (any kind) and get to know marjoram—oregano's often neglected, more subtle cousin. The key is not to wash the mushrooms in water or they'll get soggy.*

2 tablespoons olive oil
1 pound fresh mushrooms, wiped
   clean and sliced
2 tablespoons fresh marjoram
   leaves, chopped
Salt and pepper to taste

Heat the olive oil in a large sauté pan over high heat and sauté the mushrooms until lightly done—very lightly browned and still meaty, not limp. Turn off the heat, season with marjoram and salt and pepper, toss, and serve.

## TIP

*Don't wash mushrooms with water—they get soggy. Dry-clean them, wiping the dirt off with a lightly dampened paper towel.*

# Simple Eggplant

*Prepare this eggplant dish to use as an addition to stir-frys, on pizza, or as a side dish.*

1 eggplant
1 tablespoon soy sauce
1 tablespoon balsamic vinegar
1 tablespoon olive oil

Preheat toaster oven to 400°F.

Wash the outside of the eggplant, pierce it with a fork a few times, and cook in a microwave for about 5 minutes, until slightly soft. Remove the eggplant from the microwave, quarter it lengthwise, and place pieces skin side down on the baking tray of a toaster oven. Drizzle the eggplant with the soy sauce, the vinegar, and then the olive oil. Bake in preheated toaster oven until browned, about 20 minutes.

 **TIP**

*If a vegetable is on sale it's probably in season and it's a good time to use it.*

# Root-Vegetable Crepes

*A throwback to old macro days. Root vegetables keep you grounded. Eat them often, with or without the crepes.*

**For the root-vegetable filling:**

*1 large sweet potato or yam,*
  *washed and diced*
*2 carrots, washed and diced*
*1 large onion, peeled and chopped*
*1 turnip, washed and diced*
*1 baking potato, washed and diced*
*3 tablespoons soy sauce (more or*
  *less, use low-sodium)*
*2 tablespoons sake (optional)*
*1 3-inch piece fresh ginger root,*
  *thinly sliced*
*2 to 3 cups water or stock*
*2 tablespoons white flour*
*1 tablespoon vegetable oil*

Preheat the oven to 400°F

Put all the vegetables in a large baking pan (don't pile them up too deep). Add the soy sauce, sake (if desired), and ginger to the pan. Pour water or stock over the vegetables until they are just peaking out of the liquid (not quite covered). Add the flour and mix the whole thing up to blend. Drizzle with vegetable oil and bake for 50 minutes to 1 hour. Before filling crepes, pick out the ginger pieces.

**For the crepes:**
*1 cup white flour*
*2 eggs*
*1 1/2 cups water*
*1/2 teaspoon or less salt*
*Chopped scallions, as garnish*

Combine all the ingredients (except scallions) for the crepes and mix well with a wire whisk.

Heat a nonstick skillet over medium heat until it's very hot. (Swipe the pan with a paper towel dabbed in vegetable oil before every other crepe.) Add a small ladleful of batter to the pan. Swish it around to distribute the batter and make the crepe as thin as possible (you can pour some out if necessary). Cook for 45 seconds to 1 minute on the first side (as soon as the edges curl you can lift and turn—crepes should be lightly done). Turn crepe over and continue to cook for 10 to 20 seconds. Stack the finished crepe on a plate. Repeat until batter is used up (this recipe makes 10 to 12 filled crepes).

Fill each crepe with root-vegetable filling, roll, and top with a bit of the pan sauce. Garnish with chopped scallions.

# Fire-Roasted Eggplant Timbales

*Cute on the plate and scrumptious on the palate. Fire-roast at home for an "out in the woods" experience.*

2 eggplants
2 red bell peppers
2 tablespoons olive oil
1 large onion, finely chopped
2 teaspoons balsamic vinegar
1 tablespoon soy sauce
Salt and pepper

Fire up four gas burners to low-medium heat and set the eggplants and peppers directly on the burner grate. If you have an electric stove, roast the peppers and the egg-plants in the oven at 450°F for about 40 minutes and proceed the best you can as follows: When they burn, give them a turn (use a tong or a fork). Continue to cook until they are blackened all around, about 20 minutes.

Place the blackened veggies in a paper bag and close it up. (This helps to sweat off the skins.)

Heat the olive oil in a frying pan and sauté the onion until lightly browned. Turn off the heat and add the soy sauce and balsamic vinegar to the pan.

Preheat oven to 400°F.

Remove the burnt veggies from the bag and wash the skins off under gently running water. Do the best you can with the eggplants. Cut the peppers into small squares and the eggplant into bite-sized chunks, put them in a large bowl, and salt and pepper them lightly. Add the saucy sautéed onion to the bowl and mix it up.

Grease some Pyrex custard cups with olive oil and press as much of the veggie mixture as you can into each one. If you want to get fancy, arrange the pepper squares or sprigs of fresh herbs on the bottom of the custard cup. Place the filled custard cups in a baking dish and fill the dish with enough water to reach halfway up the sides of the custard cups. Bake in preheated oven for 40 minutes. Remove and allow to cool. Turn upside down and bang out onto individual plates to serve.

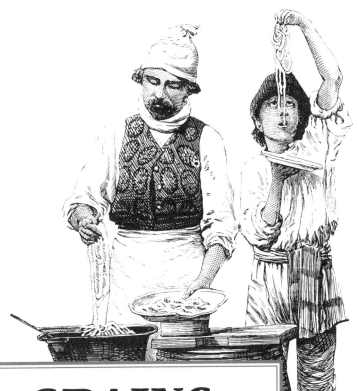

# PASTA, GRAINS, AND POTATOES

# Yakisoba

*This is a quick-cooking dish that really sticks to your ribs. Pan-fried buckwheat noodles. (Don't overcook the noodles or they'll get mushy.)*

*You can also cook this dish with udon, soba's whole wheat cousin.*

8 ounces soba noodles (buckwheat)
I tablespoon sesame or peanut oil
4 slices fresh ginger
I onion, sliced thin
I large carrot, cut into long
   matchsticks
I cup shredded cabbage
I clove garlic, minced
2 tablespoons soy sauce
Chopped scallion greens

Bring 6 quarts of water to a rapid boil. Add the noodles to the pot and cook, stirring occasionally, until al dente, 9 to 12 minutes. Rinse with cool water to stop cooking and set aside.

Heat the oil in a large sauté pan or a wok, add the ginger and the onion, and sauté for a few minutes. Add the carrot and cabbage, stir, and fry for a few more minutes. Add the garlic and the noodles and continue stirring and frying. (If the pan gets dry and things are sticking, add water or stock to the pan I tablespoon at a time.)

When the vegetables become tender and the noodles are slightly browned, add the soy sauce to the pan and continue to stir and fry for a minute or so. Spill onto a large platter and serve, garnished with chopped scallions.

*Trying to get funding for a PBS cooking show is harder than Chinese algebra. I feel like Virginia Woolf or somebody the way I'm always writing letters. I wish I didn't want to do the show so badly, but the idea of inviting a million people into my kitchen (without costly structural changes) thrills me to death—Come on in and stir-fry awhile, meet my favorite implements, check out these ingredients. I'd like to have a fireplace and an observation bar for guests on the show. We'll share ideas, cut the cake, and have a glass. Y'all come back now, y'hear.*

# Mongolian Flatbread

*A chewy comfort food and side starch that goes well with saucy entrees. I like to serve these pancake-style with Mongolian BBQ (p. 108). Give your guests a chance to flip.*

*You can use this same batter to make English muffins (see below).*

3 cups unbleached white flour
2 teaspoons sweetener
1 package dry yeast
2 teaspoons salt, or to taste
1 ¼ cups slightly warm milk or soy milk
1 cup slightly warm water
Vegetable oil, for frying

Combine the flour, sweetener, yeast, and salt together in a large mixing bowl and make a well in the center. Add the water and milk and whisk vigorously, about 5 minutes, to make a very smooth batter. Cover the bowl with plastic wrap and let sit in a warm place for about 1 hour (surface should be bubbled).

Whisk the batter for another minute and it's ready to go.

Set the oven on warm for later. Put a teaspoon or so (more for a fried-dough effect) of vegetable oil in a non-stick frying pan, place over medium-low heat, and fry a ladleful of batter at a time for a few minutes on each side, until well browned, keeping the pan covered while frying. Place finished cakes in the oven to keep warm.

**To make English muffins:**
Instead of using ladlefuls, place round, greased, metal cookie cutters in the well-oiled frying pan and pour the batter into the center of the cookie cutters to fill. Fry for a few minutes on each side—flipping cookie cutter and batter together. Keep a growing stack of griddle cakes warm in the oven until ready to serve.

These freeze well and can be warmed in the oven.

# Flat-Crust Pizza Dough

*Keep these simple ingredients and a jar of red sauce on hand for fresh pizza anytime. Get creative with toppings. Rent a movie.*

3 cups unbleached white flour
1 package dry yeast
1 teaspoon salt
1 teaspoon sweetener
1 cup lukewarm water
2 tablespoons olive oil

Thoroughly combine the flour, yeast, salt, and sweetener together in a large glass bowl. Make a well in the dough, add the water and the oil, and mix.

Spread some flour on a work surface and knead the dough mixture, adding small amounts of flour as necessary to make dough soft and smooth. This should take about 5 minutes. Put the dough back in the bowl and cover it tightly with plastic wrap or a damp towel. Let it sit in a warm place for about 1 hour until it doubles in size.

Punch down the dough (to take the air out) and cut it in half. Knead one piece at a time for just a few minutes on a floured surface and form each into a ball.

Using a rolling pin or a bottle, roll the ball of dough out into a flat circle to fit a pizza pan. Roll from the inside out and repeat as needed to get a uniform thickness. The circle of dough should be about $1/8$-inch thick at this point. Repeat with the remaining ball of dough. Preheat the oven to 425°F.

The crusts are now ready to top with your favorites.

Bake in preheated oven until crisp and browned on the edges, about 15 to 20 minutes.

*A pizza shell is an empty palette. Use your imagination, or use the usual. I generally start with sauce, then cheese, then veggies, then more cheese, then herbs and a drizzle of olive oil.*

# Sicilian Pizza Dough

*Semolina flour gives this dough a delicious nutty aroma. Use your choice of toppings.*

2 cups unbleached white flour
1 cup semolina flour
1 teaspoon salt
1 package dry yeast
1 cup warm water
2 tablespoons olive oil
1 egg
Cornmeal, for dusting

Combine both flours, the salt, and the yeast in a large glass bowl. Make a well in the flour mixture and add the water, oil, and egg. Mix well with your hands. Turn the dough out onto a floured surface and knead for a few minutes, until smooth. Sprinkle a 9- by 12-inch baking pan with cornmeal to prevent sticking. Roll the dough out to fill the pan, cover with plastic wrap, and let rise for about 1 hour. Top pizza dough with whatever you like and bake for about 30 minutes in an oven preheated to 400°F.

*I teach a class called "Doughs I Can Deal With." Pizza, English muffins, gnocchi, and quick breads are doughs worth dealing with because the final product is more than worth the time and effort spent in the kitchen. I don't understand why someone would be willing to spend four or five hours slaving away to produce something you can buy for three dollars. Why not try my quick doughs? They give the illusion of slaving with stellar results. If you really want to impress someone, powder your face with flour before serving the completed product. This will create the effect of kitchen martyrdom.*

# Dilled Rice

*Here's a green one with a Russian feel. The rice and potatoes groove together texturally.*

1 tablespoon olive oil
1 onion, diced
1 cup peeled and cubed potato
2 cups white rice
2 cloves garlic, chopped
4 cups water or stock
Salt and pepper to taste
1 bunch dill, stems trimmed and
   chopped

Heat the oil in a 3- or 4-quart pot that has a tight-fitting lid, add the onion, and sauté. When the onion starts to brown add the potato, the rice, and the garlic and continue to stir while frying for a few minutes.

Add the water or stock, salt and pepper to taste, and dill and bring to a boil. Lower the heat to a simmer, cover, and let cook until all the liquid has been absorbed, about 20 to 25 minutes. Let the rice sit for a few minutes before serving.

# Gnocchi

*A doughy dish I can deal with. Fun, easy, and delicious. Don't try to make love after you eat a plateful of these dumplings.*

3 pounds baking potatoes, washed and
　　left whole
2 eggs
1 teaspoon salt
Dash of pepper
4 cups unbleached white flour

Boil the potatoes until soft, about 25 to 30 minutes. Drain and allow to cool.

Put a large pot of salted water on to boil.

Mash or rice the potatoes into a large mixing bowl.

In a separate, small bowl, beat the eggs and add the salt and pepper to them. Mix the eggs into the potatoes and whip smooth with a wire whisk.

Add 3 cups of the flour to the potatoes, stirring it in 1 cup at a time. The dough should be soft and smooth but not overworked. After adding the third cup of flour, take the dough out of the bowl and place on a floured work surface. Continue to knead gently for about 5 to 10 minutes, adding flour as needed to make a soft, dry (but not sticky) dough.

Pull off small handfuls of the dough, shape into balls in the palm of your hand, and roll each ball into a rope about 1-inch thick. Cut the ropes at a slant, making little $1/2$-inch "pillows," or gnocchi.

Boil a few dozen gnocchi at a time in rapidly boiling water. When they rise to the top, let them cook for 1 or 2 minutes more. Strain and serve hot with red sauce, creamy sauce, herb sauce, or whatever. For different-flavored gnocchi, try adding roasted red pepper, chives, or other fresh herbs to the dough.

# Rosemary Roasted Potatoes

*Any potatoes will do for this recipe, but I like the little red ones.*

2 pounds potatoes, sliced or
    quartered
2 tablespoons fresh rosemary
    leaves, chopped
2 tablespoons olive oil
Salt and pepper to taste

Preheat oven to 450°F.

Combine all ingredients thoroughly—*grease them taters!* Place potato pieces in single-file rows on a nonstick cookie sheet and bake in preheated oven for 40 to 50 minutes, adding a few tablespoons of water to pan during cooking to prevent sticking.

# Greek Spinach-Rice

*Spinach and rice. Nice.*

1 tablespoon olive oil, or more
1 onion, chopped
2 cloves garlic, chopped
1 pound spinach, washed and
    chopped
2 cups white rice
2 tomatoes, chopped
1 bunch fresh dill, chopped
4 cups water or stock

Heat the olive oil in a large saucepan with a tight-fitting lid. Add the onion and the garlic and sauté until the onion is lightly browned. Add the spinach and the rice and continue to sauté for 2 to 3 minutes.

Add the rest of the ingredients and bring the pot to a boil. Reduce the heat to a low simmer and cover the pot. Cook until all the liquid is absorbed and the rice is tender, about 20 minutes.

# Lemon Herbed Rice

*Fresh herbs and a fine olive oil can make rice talk. Try this dish using either leftover or freshly cooked rice. Serve it hot as a side dish or cold as a salad.*

1 tablespoon lemon juice
1 tablespoon or more olive oil
1 tablespoon chopped fresh parsley
1 tablespoon chopped fresh mint
   (or thyme)
Salt and pepper to taste
$1/2$ teaspoon lemon zest
2 cups cooked rice

Place the lemon juice in a large bowl and whisk in the oil. Add the herbs, salt and pepper, and lemon zest. Break up the rice as you add it to the bowl and mix well. *Voila.*

*Most people (myself included) eat the same dishes over and over again at home. We'll have the noodle thing on Monday and the rice thing Tuesday, and so on and so forth. I guess we are creatures of habit, but I like to think of myself as more adventurous than that. Maybe life outside the kitchen is adventurous enough? Where the road "out there" twists and turns and stops nobody knows. The kitchen is the place for comfort and the known. It takes courage to change something so close to home, but when we do, it expands our world.*

# Vegetarian Pad Thai

*The most famous of Thai dishes is easy to make at home. Add bite-sized chunks of boneless chicken or peeled shrimp (or both) in place of the mushroom for a carnivorous version.*

$1/2$ pound flat white rice noodles

1 tablespoon white vinegar

3 tablespoons fish sauce

$1 1/2$ tablespoons or more sweetener

1 tablespoon tomato paste

$1/4$ teaspoon black pepper

1 tablespoon peanut or canola oil

1 onion, chopped

1 green bell pepper, chopped

2 cloves garlic, chopped

1 carrot, cut into matchsticks

$1/2$ pound portabello mushrooms,
    cut into $1/2$-inch square chunks

1 cup bean sprouts

$1/4$ cup crushed dry-roasted peanuts

Cilantro leaves for garnish

Bring a large pot of water to a boil and turn off the heat. Put the noodles into the pot and let sit for 5 to 10 minutes, checking often for desired doneness (al dente). When the noodles are done, rinse them in cold water and set aside.

In a small bowl, mix the vinegar, fish sauce, sweetener, tomato paste, and black pepper.

Heat the oil in a wok or large frying pan. Add the onion and the green pepper and sauté for a few minutes. Add the garlic, carrot matchsticks, and mushrooms and continue to sauté until the vegetables are tender and slightly caramelized (browned).

Add the sauce mixture to the pan and cook for 1 minute. Add the noodles and a few tablespoons of water and toss to mix thoroughly. Turn off the heat, add the bean sprouts to the noodles, and toss lightly. Garnish with peanuts and cilantro and serve.

# Whole-Spice Pilaf

*A clever use of whole spices makes this vegetarian side dish super satisfying.*

2 tablespoons or less olive oil
1 onion, chopped
1 1/2 cups rice
3 cups water or stock
2 3-inch-long cinnamon sticks
3 bay leaves, crumbled
20 whole peppercorns
8 cardamom pods, cracked
1/2 teaspoon turmeric
Salt to taste
1 green bell pepper, sliced very thin
1 red bell pepper, sliced very thin
Whole sprigs of cilantro

In a 3-quart pot, heat the oil and sauté the onion until lightly browned. Add the rice and continue to stir-fry. When the rice starts to brown, add the stock or water and all the spices and bring the pot to a boil. Turn the heat down to a simmer, cover the pot tightly, and cook until all the liquid is absorbed, about 20 minutes. Turn off the heat and let the pot sit, covered, for at least 5 minutes more to continue steaming.

Toss the hot rice in a large bowl with the green and red pepper slices and garnish with cilantro.

*Using whole spices in a dish is cool, even if you have to spit one out on occasion. You know what you're eating when you bite into a peppercorn or a cardamom pod. In this world of uncertainty and gray areas, it's refreshing to come across anything that knows exactly what it is. It screams out,* I'm here to flavor this dish; you have a problem with that, don't use me! Go get one of those cans that have been sitting in your kitchen cabinet for five years. They don't have any flavor left because all their essential oils have dissipated, while mine are fertile and strong. *Using whole spices is kind of macho.*

# Pressure-Cooked Brown Rice with Wheat Berries

*Macro days are here again. I don't like the texture of brown rice if it's boiled, but pressure-cooked brown rice is fluffy and chewy. Leftover rice is great for a stuffing.*

2 cups short-grain brown rice
$^1/_2$ cup wheat berries
4 cups water
Salt to taste

Combine all ingredients in a pressure cooker, cover, seal, and bring to pressure. Lower heat and continue to pressure-cook for 40 minutes. Remove the pressure cooker from the heat, place it in the sink, and run cool water over the edge to bring down the pressure. Open, fluff, and serve.

*Brown rice is the most balanced (pH-wise) food in nature. That's why macrobiotics' diets are 50 to 70 percent grain. That's a lot of carbs. The new Zone Diet recommends eating carbs in tiny amounts, as a condiment, like salsa. If the Zoners and the macros had a picnic you'd have a Jack Sprat situation. They might even get along if they could agree to disagree.*

# Eliopita

*This olive-batter bread is popular in Cyprus. Serve it hot with slices of ripe red tomatoes as a side dish or appetizer. Leftover eliopita is a great stuffing for chicken. (This dish is a lot better than it sounds, really).*

3$^1/_2$ cups unbleached white flour

1 heaping tablespoon baking powder

1 teaspoon salt

2 cups warm water

1 cup olive oil

$^1/_2$ pound Calamata olives, pitted and chopped

2 tablespoons chopped fresh mint leaves

1 medium onion, chopped fine

Preheat the oven to 350°F.

Combine the flour, baking powder, and salt in a large mixing bowl. Slowly mix in the warm water and the olive oil to make a batter. Do not overmix. Fold in the olives, mint, and onion.

Grease 2 pie pans with olive oil. Use a rubber spatula to scrape the batter into the greased baking pans and smooth it out. Bake the breads in the preheated oven for 35 to 45 minutes, until lightly browned and firm to the touch.

# TIP

*Measure out a tablespoon of flour and put it in the palm of your hand. Then do the same with a teaspoon of flour. Remember how each looks and feels. Now you can measure without measuring. Use your hands as much as possible to get more involved in the process of cooking.*

# Arroz à la Mexicana

*Add chunks of zucchini and shrimp or chicken to make a meal out of this simple but satisfying rice dish. Serve with Baked Fish, Yucatan Style (p. 96) or Grilled Chicken, Yucatan Style (p. 114).*

1 tablespoon or more olive oil

1 large onion, chopped

4 cloves garlic, minced

2 cups long-grain white rice

2 cups canned peeled tomatoes
    (Mexican-flavored if possible)

3 cups water or stock

Salt and pepper to taste

$^1/_2$ cup carrot rounds

$^1/_2$ cup frozen peas

Parsley or cilantro leaves

Heat the oil in a 3-quart pot that has a tight-fitting lid. Add the onion and sauté for a few minutes. Add the garlic and the rice and continue to sauté until the rice turns golden. Add the tomatoes, water or stock, and salt and pepper and bring the pot to a boil. Turn the heat down to a simmer, add the carrot rounds, cover the pot, and cook until the liquid is gone, about 20 minutes.

Turn off the heat, add the frozen peas, cover again, and let sit for a few minutes. Serve garnished with parsley or cilantro.

# TIP

*Don't refrigerate prepared grain dishes. Cold air dries them out. Make just enough to last a day or two and leave it out.*

# Mushroom Lo Mein

*Lo mein means "tossed noodles," so get tossing. Fresh Chinese noodles are available in Oriental food markets. If you can't find them, use fresh linguini. Vary the vegetables or add chicken or shrimp for variety.*

12 ounces fresh Chinese noodles
1 tablespoon or more peanut or
   canola oil
1-inch piece of ginger, minced
3 or 4 cloves garlic, minced
1 bunch scallions, chopped
$^1/_2$ pound mushrooms, wiped clean
   and sliced
1 carrot, cut into matchsticks
2 tablespoons soy sauce
Dash of black pepper
$^1/_4$ cup stock or water
Scallion greens, slivered, as garnish

Cook the noodles al dente, strain, and set aside.

Heat the oil in a large frying pan or a wok, add the ginger, and sauté for a minute. Add the garlic and the vegetables and stir-fry for 1 or 2 minutes. Add the noodles, the soy sauce, and the pepper and continue to stir-fry for another minute.

Add the stock to the pan 1 tablespoon at a time while stirring and frying for another few minutes. Serve garnished with slivered scallions.

*Noodles were invented because of an energy crisis in ancient China. A whole grain (wheat, corn, rice, etc.) takes a hell of a lot of energy to cook (boil for 30 minutes to 1 hour), but if you bust it up into flour and make noodles it cooks pretty quickly (boil for 5 to 12 minutes). When you consider the amount of wood necessary to actually boil a large pot of water, the difference in cooking time is substantial. Think about it the next time you have Oodles of Noodles for lunch.*

# Polenta Puttanesca

*There's a story behind this sauce. Roman housewives are "fooling around" while their husbands are at work. They return home just before their husbands and make a quick sauce that tastes like it took all day to prepare. Long-cooked flavor in a short time. Everyday delight.*

**For the polenta:**

*2 cups water*
*¹/₂ cup cornmeal*
*Salt to taste*

Bring the water to a boil in a large saucepan. Gradually add the cornmeal, stirring constantly with a wire whisk. Lower the temperature and continue to cook while stirring until the polenta is thick and creamy, about 25 minutes. Pour into greased pie plates and refrigerate for later use. To serve, cut into wedges and sauté in olive oil.

**For the puttanesca sauce:**

*2 tablespoons olive oil*
*4 anchovy filets*
*4 cloves garlic, minced*
*1 28-ounce can peeled tomatoes, drained and chopped*
*3 tablespoons chopped fresh parsley*
*1 teaspoon dry oregano (or 1 tablespoon fresh)*
*2 tablespoons capers, drained*
*12 olives, pitted and chopped*
*¹/₂ teaspoon or more red pepper flakes*

Heat the olive oil and the anchovies in a large frying pan until the anchovies begin to dissolve. Add the garlic and continue to sauté for a few seconds (don't let it brown). Add the tomatoes and all the other ingredients, bring to a simmer, and cook for 10 to 15 minutes.

This sauce works with grilled fish or chicken as well as pasta.

# Paella

*The classic Spanish rice dish—the way I like it.*
*    Boil a lobster for 10 minutes and use the boiling water for stock in the recipe. Add the lobster to the pot with the clams and mussels and use it to make a dramatic presentation.*

2 tablespoons or less olive oil
2 chicken legs, bone in
2 chicken thighs, bone in
4 turkey sausages
1 large onion, chopped
1 large green pepper, diced large
2 or 3 cloves garlic, chopped
1 1/2 cups short-grain white rice (I
    like sushi rice or arborio)
1 cup white wine
2 cups stock or water
Pinch saffron
Salt and pepper to taste
1 large ripe tomato, chopped
2 pounds shellfish, in any combination:
    Mussels
    Clams
    Peeled shrimp
1 roasted red pepper, sliced in strips and
    marinated in vinegar, as
    garnish
Chopped parsley, as garnish
Lemon wedges, as garnish

Heat the oil in a large frying pan, cast-iron Dutch oven, or a wok that has a cover. Add the chicken and begin to brown it. Add the sausage and continue to cook until the chicken is very well browned (you can pour some of the grease off now if desired). Add the onion and the green pepper and cook until the onion starts to brown. Add the garlic and continue to sauté for a minute. Add the rice and toss it around until well coated with pan juices and slightly browned (brown is the name of the game here). Add the wine to the pot and stir, toss, and let bubble.

Add the stock, saffron, and salt and pepper and bring the pot to a boil. Reduce the heat to a simmer and cover. When the water is almost halfway down through the rice, add the tomato and the shellfish to the pot. Cover and continue to cook until all the liquid is absorbed, the rice is tender, and the shellfish are cooked (mussels and clams open, shrimp pink).

Put the pot on the table family style and garnish with strips of marinated red pepper (pimentos), lemon wedges, and parsley.

 **TIP**

*Wrap your leftovers in a tortilla and,* voila, *you have lunch.*

# Pasta, My Way

*Move over Frank.*

*1 large eggplant*
*Balsamic vinegar for drizzling, plus 2*
*tablespoons for the sauté*
*Soy sauce for drizzling, plus 2*
*tablespoons for the sauté*
*Olive oil for drizzling, plus about 1*
*tablespoon for sautéeing*
*Freshly ground black pepper*
*$1/2$ pound pasta (any kind but the*
*long ones)*
*1 onion, coarsely chopped*
*1 red bell pepper, coarsely chopped*
*1 carrot*
*$1/2$ bunch broccoli or broccoli rabe*
*$1/2$ cup sun-dried tomatoes, covered*
*with water in a small bowl and*
*microwaved for 2 minutes*
*2 cloves minced garlic, optional*

Poke a few holes in the eggplant and microwave for 5 minutes. Quarter it lengthwise and drizzle with balsamic vinegar, then soy sauce, then olive oil. Sprinkle with a grind of black pepper and broil it in the toaster oven (or conventional oven) until well browned, about 20 minutes. Dice the eggplant into 1-inch squares and set aside. Boil the pasta and set aside (reserve some of the pasta water, you'll see why later).

Heat a large frying pan or a wok over medium-high heat (wait until it's close to smoking) and add the chopped onion (hear the sizzle). When the onion begins to brown, add the red pepper, the carrot, and the broccoli and continue to fry and stir. If the pan gets dry add some of the pasta water 1 tablespoon at a time. (If you add too much water you'll be simmering in liquid and lowering the temperature in the pan.) Only add as much as you need to keep it a sauté. When the veggies are almost tender, add the pasta, the sun-dried tomatoes, the garlic if desired, the roasted eggplant, the 2 tablespoons balsamic, the 2 tablespoons soy sauce, and a few grinds of pepper and continue to stir and fry. Add more pasta water as necessary to keep it juicy (but not too much, this is more of a coating than a sauce). Cook until all ingredients are well coated and the pasta is lightly pan-seared.

Taste. If you like it saltier, add more soy sauce. If you like it more on the tangy side, add more balsamic or serve with a squeeze of lemon.

# Southtown Corn Bread

*A Boston favorite. Try sweetening with maple syrup for a real down-home feel.*

**Dry ingredients:**

1 1/4 cups cornmeal
1 1/4 cups unbleached white flour
2 1/2 teaspoons baking powder
1 teaspoon or less salt
1/2 cup corn kernels, fresh or frozen,
    optional

**Wet ingredients:**

3 tablespoons unrefined corn oil
2 eggs (or 3 egg whites)
2 to 4 tablespoons sweetener
1 cup soy milk, rice milk, or milk milk

Preheat the oven to 350°F. Grease a pie plate, muffin tins, or a loaf pan with corn oil.

Combine all the dry ingredients (except the corn kernels) in a large mixing bowl and whisk to sift.

In a separate bowl, combine all the wet ingredients and whisk well. Add the wet ingredients to the dry and mix gently with a rubber spatula or large spoon until well blended. Add the kernels at this point if desired. Pour the batter, which should be thick but just about pourable with a little help from your spatula, into the greased baking dish of choice. Bake in preheated oven for 20 to 35 minutes depending on the depth of the baking dish. Serve hot.

# Pineapple Shrimp-Fried Rice

*This recipe works with noodles as well (use $^1/_2$ pound cooked rice or wheat noodles). Fresh pineapple is best but canned is okay too.*

1 tablespoon Thai curry paste (I like
   yellow for this dish)
$^3/_4$ cup coconut milk
1 onion, chopped
1 red bell pepper, chopped
1 teaspoon sweetener
2 tablespoons fish sauce
1 teaspoon lemon zest
1 pound medium shrimp, shelled
   and deveined (or chunks of
   chicken)
4 cups cooked jasmine rice
1 $^1/_2$ cups pineapple chunks
6 basil leaves, shredded

Place a wok over high heat, get it hot, and sauté the curry paste with 2 tablespoons of the coconut milk for about a minute. Add the onion and pepper and continue to sauté for a few minutes. Add the rest of the coconut milk, the sweetener, fish sauce, and lemon zest and bring to a boil.

Add the shrimp, rice, and pineapple and stir-fry until the coconut milk has cooked down a bit (it shouldn't be too wet, just a little sticky), the shrimp is cooked, and all the ingredients are well blended. Serve garnished with shredded basil leaves.

# TIP

*There are 40,000 varieties of rice but they're all cooked the same way: 2 cups of water to 1 cup of rice. Put the water and rice in a pot, turn up the heat, and bring the pot to a boil. Add a little salt, turn the heat down to low to simmer, cover, and cook until all the liquid is absorbed by the rice.*

# Cardamom Pilaf

*If you can't find whole cardamom pods, use 1 teaspoon of powdered. If you don't like cooked nuts, use them uncooked as a garnish or leave them out. It's up to you.*

1 tablespoon or more olive oil
1 onion, chopped
$1/4$ cup pine nuts
2 cups white rice, any kind will do
4 cups water or chicken stock
10 cardamom pods, cracked
3 cinnamon sticks (or a heaping
   $1/2$ teaspoon)
12 peppercorns
Salt to taste
8 dried figs (not too hard—if they're
   really hard add water and
   microwave for a minute),
   chopped
Chopped parsley

Heat the olive oil over high heat in a good-sized saucepan that has a tight-fitting lid, add the onion, and sauté until it starts to brown. Add the pine nuts and the rice and continue to sauté until the nuts smell sweet and the rice gets a bit golden (don't let anything get stuck to the bottom of the pot). Add the water (or chicken stock), the spices and salt, and the figs and bring the pot to a full boil. Reduce the heat to a low simmer and cover the pot. Cook until all the water has evaporated, about 20 to 25 minutes, and let stand covered for a few minutes before serving. Garnish with chopped parsley.

# Veggie Jambalaya

*More veggies is "more better" (As you can tell, I love this expression.) If fresh tomatoes are not available you could use canned peeled tomatoes (chopped).*

1 tablespoon or more olive oil
1 large onion, chopped
1 green pepper, chopped
2 stalks celery, diced
2 or 3 cloves garlic, minced
1 tablespoon flour, optional (I'll explain later)
2 cups chopped fresh ripe tomatoes
2 bay leaves, broken up
1 teaspoon dried thyme
1 $1/2$ cups long-grain white rice (or arborio)
2 $1/2$ cups stock or water
Salt and pepper to taste
1 cup string beans, cut into 2-inch pieces
2 carrots, sliced into fairly thin rounds
Chopped parsley

Heat the oil in a large saucepan (that has a cover) and sauté the onion, pepper, and celery. When the onion starts to brown, add the garlic and continue to sauté for another minute. For a nice touch in terms of texture, you may choose to add the flour now. (This step is optional because it requires a lot of watching. It's very easy to burn the bottom of the pot and ruin the dish if the flour sticks, and flour tends to cling in this situation.) If you decide to go with the flour option (it's up to you) add the flour and stir-fry until vegetables are coated and flour is light brown. Watch closely and scrape the bottom now and again. Add the tomatoes, their juice, the bay leaves, and thyme and stir it up. When it bubbles, add the rice and the stock or water and bring the pot to a boil. Add salt and pepper, turn the pot down to a low simmer, and cover. Continue to cook for 7 or 8 minutes.

Rest the carrots and string beans on top of the rice, cover, and continue to cook until all the liquid is absorbed, about 15 to 20 minutes. Turn off the heat and let stand for a few minutes. Serve garnished with chopped parsley.

## TIP

*Get a vegetable brush. It'll save you from doing some peeling and the left-on skin has nutritional value.*

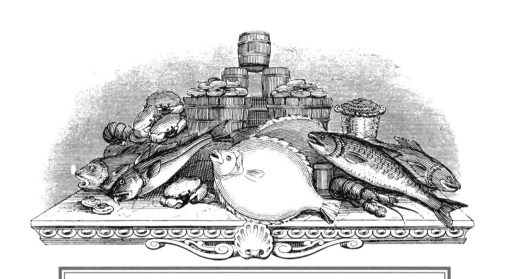

# SEAFOOD

# Panang Curried Salmon with Asparagus

*You can make this dish with red or yellow curry paste as well. It's seriously delicious.*

2 tablespoons Panang curry paste

1 14-ounce can coconut milk

1 onion, diced

1 tablespoon Thai fish sauce, or
   more to taste

1 tablespoon sweetener, or more to
   taste

1 pound fresh asparagus, ends
   trimmed

1 pound fresh salmon filet, skinned
   and boned, cut into 4 sections

1 bunch fresh basil leaves

1 ripe tomato, diced

Fry the curry paste with a few tablespoons of the coconut milk over high heat in a wok or a large frying pan that has a lid. Stir and fry for 1 or 2 minutes. Add the onion and continue to stir-fry for a few more minutes. Add the rest of the coconut milk, the fish sauce, and the sweetener and bring to a low boil. Reduce the heat to a simmer and lay the asparagus stalks side by side in the sauce to form a rack for the salmon.

Place the salmon on top of the asparagus, cover the pan, and cook for 7 to 10 minutes, checking the salmon for desired doneness. Garnish with fresh basil leaves and diced tomato and serve with jasmine or white rice.

*When I go out to eat, I like to be taken care of. I always order something I would never make at home. Something really time-consuming, complicated, exotic, or made with equipment I don't have in my kitchen. I relish being attended to. Being taken care of can never be overrated. It appeals to the inner prince or princess in each of us. Remember how special you are the next time you're in a restaurant, and dare to be a little fussy.*

# Mustard-Tarragon Shark Kebabs

*Try this marinade with shellfish, swordfish, or chicken. It's a delicious way to get to know the noble tarragon.*

**For the mustard-tarragon marinade:**

2 teaspoons Dijon mustard

3 tablespoons white wine (or champagne)

2 tablespoons olive oil

1 tablespoon fresh tarragon leaves (or 1$^1/_2$ teaspoons dry)

Salt and pepper to taste

**For the shark kebabs:**

1 pound shark, cut into large, bite-sized chunks

1 zucchini, sliced into thin rounds (thick enough to skewer)

1 bell pepper, cut into chunks

Cherry tomatoes

Wooden skewers

Place all the ingredients for the mustard-tarragon marinade in a small bowl and whisk together.

Place the shark chunks and prepared veggies in a shallow glass dish or baking pan. Cover with the marinade and marinate for 1 to 2 hours in the fridge, turning to coat halfway through.

Skewer the marinated shark and veggie pieces and broil or grill for a few minutes on each side.

*Try shark for a change. It has a swordfish-like consistency at half the price. The flavor is heartier, but a robust marinade will use that to an advantage. The special someone in my life is deathly afraid of sharks and finds it empowering to eat shark.*
*"I eat shark, shark doesn't eat me" is her shark eating mantra. I say, get it where you can, girl.*

# Salmon-Corn Dumplings in Fresh Tomato Soup

*This soup can be served hot or cold. Vary the herbs for a change of taste. The dumplings are like gefilte fish, but pink. Viva la difference!*

**For the soup:**

2 tablespoons olive oil
4 shallots, chopped
12 peppercorns, crushed
4 pounds ripe tomatoes, diced
2 tablespoons tomato paste
2 tablespoons chopped fresh
   parsley
1 tablespoon fresh thyme (plus
   extra for garnish)
1 tablespoon balsamic vinegar
2 cups chicken stock

To make the soup, heat the olive oil in a heavy-bottomed saucepan and sauté the shallots until lightly browned. Add the crushed peppercorns, the tomatoes, and the tomato paste and sauté for a few more minutes. Add the stock and bring the pot to a boil. Turn the heat down to low and simmer for 15 minutes.

Add the herbs and seasonings, turn off the heat, and let sit for 5 to 10 minutes.

Puree in a food processor until smooth. Refrigerate or put back into the pot to warm.

**For the dumplings:**

2 teaspoons tomato paste
$^1/_4$ cup flour
2 eggs
2 scallions, chopped
Salt and pepper to taste
$^3/_4$ pound fresh salmon filet, skinned
   and boned, cut into chunks
$^1/_2$ cup corn kernels, fresh or frozen

To make the dumplings, put the tomato paste, flour, eggs, scallions, and salt and pepper in the work bowl of the food processor or a blender and puree. Add the salmon and continue to process until chunky smooth.

Mix in the corn kernels by hand (the batter will be slightly loose and wet).

Drop heaping spoonfuls of the batter into gently boiling water and cook for 3 to 4 minutes (not more than 4 dumplings at a time). When the dumplings float to the top they are ready.

Float the dumplings in the soup and serve hot or cold, garnished with fresh herbs.

# BBQ Salmon with Pineapple

*My favorite dish of last summer. You can substitute red bell pepper for the pineapple or use both.*

1 tablespoon olive oil
$^1/_4$ cup canned, crushed pineapple
    with its juice
2 tablespoons tomato paste
1 tablespoon molasses, or 2
    teaspoons brown sugar or
    Sucanat
1 teaspoon prepared mustard
1 heaping teaspoon chili powder
$^1/_2$ teaspoon cumin powder
Salt and pepper to taste
Few dashes Tabasco sauce
1-pound fresh salmon filet, skin and
    bones removed, cut into chunks
2 cups fresh pineapple, cut into
    bite-sized chunks (half the
    size of the salmon chunks)
Wooden skewers

Combine all ingredients except the salmon and fresh pineapple in a large bowl and mix well. Add the salmon and pineapple and let marinate for 30 minutes. Skewer, alternating between salmon and pineapple (or red bell pepper) and grill over high heat for 2 to 3 minutes on each side.

*I believe that anyone can cook. We human beings are related to foodstuffs by nature. Cooking is a way of shepherding our cousins in the animal and vegetable kingdoms into the pot. Go into the kitchen with an attitude of biblical proportions and have it your way. If it doesn't work out, remember—whether you waste it, baste it, or taste it—it's all compost at the end of the day.*

# Salmon and Crab Rolls

*Simple, elegant, and delicious Serve on Valentine's Day with a simple Red Pepper Puree (at right). You might get lucky.*

1-pound salmon filet, skin and pin
    bones removed
$1/3$ pound fresh crabmeat
2 tablespoons balsamic vinegar
1 tablespoon soy sauce
1 tablespoon olive oil
Freshly ground black pepper
Red Pepper Puree (p. 95)
Sprigs of fresh parsley or other
    herbs, as garnish

With a very sharp knife, slice the salmon filet lengthwise into 2 thin slices. Cut each slice in half again lengthwise. Roll $1/4$ of the crabmeat into a ball, wrap with a salmon slice, and secure with a toothpick. Repeat 3 more times. Lay the seafood rolls in a baking pan that can withstand the broiler. Drizzle the rolls with the vinegar, soy sauce, and oil, sprinkle with pepper, and broil for 6 to 8 minutes.

To serve, sauce the serving plate with Red Pepper Puree and place the rolls on top. Garnish with parsley or other fresh herb sprigs.

 **TIP**

*Don't buy seafood on Sunday (unless it's frozen anyway, like shrimp). Stores don't get seafood deliveries on Sundays, so it won't be fresh.*

# Red Pepper Puree

1 tablespoon olive oil, or less
2 red bell peppers, washed and chopped
1 onion, chopped
2 teaspoons soy sauce
1 tablespoon balsamic vinegar
Black pepper to taste

Sauté the onion and chopped red pepper in olive oil until lightly browned. Add the soy and balsamic to the pan and simmer for a minute. Puree in a food processor but leave it a little chunky. Add black pepper to taste.

*When I was a kid, my parents went on one of those cruises where you take a picture of the buffet table before dinner. There was a giant Alaskan King Crab in the center of the table. I couldn't wait to grow up. I had a dream about the crab: This huge crab and I were doing a wormy kind of tango on the buffet table. Beneath us, all the foodstuffs were squishing and crunching. I dipped my partner in a vase of butter (I was still eating dairy products at the time) and spoke to her between rose-clenching teeth, "Cannibalism is the height of sensuality my love, come to me now!"*

# Block Island Stew

*Use any type of seafood for variety. If you don't have shallots, use a combination of onion and garlic.*

1 teaspoon or more olive oil

2 shallots, chopped

1 cup dry white wine

$1/2$ teaspoon dry thyme

2 tablespoons finely chopped
   parsley

1 bay leaf

1 14-ounce can peeled tomatoes
   and their juice, tomatoes diced
   large

1-pound whitefish filet, cut into large
   chunks

$1/2$ pound clams or mussels, in their
   shells

Salt and pepper to taste

In a wok or large frying pan, heat the oil and sauté the chopped shallots until they begin to brown. Add the wine, thyme, parsley, and bay leaf and simmer for about 10 minutes. Add the diced tomatoes with juice and salt and pepper to taste, and simmer 10 minutes longer.

Layer the fish and shellfish over the sauce, cover, and simmer gently until the fish is cooked through and the shellfish open, about 10 minutes.

# TIP

*To encourage experimentation, keep a frozen entree on hand in case a recipe doesn't work out.*

# Baked Fish, Yucatan Style

*A delicious way to serve a whole fish. Mucho flavor from a harmony of spicy ingredients.*

Juice of 1 lemon
Juice of 1 orange
4 tablespoons olive oil
1 onion, chopped
2 cloves garlic, chopped
2 tomatoes, chopped
2 jalapeño peppers, seeded and
    chopped
$^1/_2$ teaspoon cinnamon
$^1/_2$ teaspoon ground cloves
1 tablespoon capers
$^1/_2$ cup water
Salt and pepper to taste
1 3- to 4-pound fish (try snapper, sea
    bass, or salmon), eviscerated,
    head and fins left on

Puree all ingredients (except the fish if you please), pour into a baking dish, add the fish, and marinate for about 1 hour.

Before the marinating time is up, preheat the oven to 375°F.

Bake the fish in the marinade in preheated oven for about 10 minutes per pound of fish.

*Refrigeration is overrated. Living on a farm in Guatemala, I was amazed at how little effect having no refrigerator and only a two-burner propane stove had on our lives, culinarily speaking. Most fruits and vegetables can keep for days without refrigeration. Cooked grains do not and should not be kept in the fridge. The cold dries them out. Even meat dishes and dairy products will keep for twenty-four hours or so. Having to live without modern conveniences keeps the chef in the house on his or her toes. This type of limitation gives focus. Give it a try for a fresh perspective.*

# Tandoori Trout

*A catchy name and a zinger of a sauce are the main attractions here. If you don't have all the spices, try using curry powder instead.*

4 trout, cleaned and butterflied,
   heads left on
1 onion, chopped
2 cloves garlic, chopped
1 tablespoon grated fresh ginger
2 tablespoons lime juice
1 teaspoon orange zest
Salt and pepper to taste
$1/2$ teaspoon coriander
$1/2$ teaspoon cumin
$1/2$ teaspoon cardamom
$1/2$ teaspoon fennel
$1/2$ teaspoon cinnamon
1 teaspoon paprika
$1/2$ cup coconut milk

Mix all ingredients (except the fish) together to make a marinade. Put about $1/3$ of the marinade in the bottom of a baking dish and place the trout in the dish in a single layer. Cover the trout with the rest of the marinade and refrigerate for 30 minutes to 1 hour.

Before the marinating time is up, preheat oven to 400°F.

Bake the fish in the marinade in preheated oven for 15 to 20 minutes until fish is browned but still moist.

# Parchment-Baked Fish Filet with Spicy Cilantro Pesto

*Try this with a green rice dish (see Dilled Rice, p. 70, and Greek Spinach-Rice, p. 73) and a green salad. Green, green, green.*

1-pound white fish filet (try ocean cat-
    fish, cod, haddock, sea bass, etc.)

$^1/_4$ cup pine nuts

2 tablespoons olive oil

$^1/_2$ cup cilantro leaves

1 jalapeño pepper, seeded and
    chopped

2 cloves garlic, minced

2 tablespoons lime juice

Salt and pepper to taste

1 piece parchment paper (or tin
    foil), 18 inches long

Preheat oven to 400°F. Sauté the pine nuts in the olive oil over low heat until golden brown.

Place the sautéed pine nuts and the cilantro, jalapeño, garlic, lime juice, and salt and pepper in a food processor and puree.

Place the fish in the center of the parchment paper (or tin foil) and cover with the pine nut puree.

Fold the paper or foil to seal and make a packet with closed ends. Bake in preheated oven for 15 to 20 minutes.

*Growing up I figured that if I ordered the most expensive thing on the menu at a restaurant it should be pretty good. I got the reputation of being a gourmet early in life, but it was really a function of economics. Now that I'm paying the bill, I'm much more discriminating, financially. I weigh the gourmet value of the meal against the cost. I analyze the ratio of the salubrious to the sapid. I calculate gastronomic pleasure received against funds depleted. And you know what, like any obsession, it's always worth it. When I'm in a restaurant, I'm like a kid in a candy store. Cost be damned—let's feast!*

# Swordfish à la Turk

*Use any firm steak fish or boneless chicken for this recipe.*

1 medium onion, chopped
$1/4$ cup fresh lemon juice
2 tablespoons olive oil
2 bay leaves, crumbled
Salt and pepper to taste
1 pound swordfish, cut into
   2-inch chunks
1 red bell pepper, cut into bite-sized
   squares
Bamboo skewers

In a food processor, puree the onion, lemon juice, oil, bay leaves, and salt and pepper to a saucy consistency.

Marinate the swordfish chunks and the red pepper pieces in the sauce for 30 minutes.

Skewer the fish and red pepper and grill or broil for a few minutes on each side.

# Trout with Red Wine, Rosemary, and Mint

*A delicious blend of distinct flavors make this simple dish a stand-out. Serve with Eggplant Salad (p. 31) and Rosemary Roasted Potatoes (p. 72) for a real flavorfest.*

2 tablespoons olive oil

I clove garlic, minced

I tablespoon chopped fresh
    rosemary leaves

Salt and pepper to taste

$^1/_2$ cup red wine

4 trout (about $^2/_3$ pound each),
    cleaned and butterflied, heads
    left on

I tablespoon or more chopped
    fresh mint leaves

Preheat oven to 425°F.

Combine the oil, garlic, rosemary, and salt and pepper. Place the fish in a baking dish and pour the oil mixture over it. Pour the wine into the dish, surrounding the fish. Place fish in preheated oven and bake for about 15 minutes. The fish should be lightly browned on top but still moist inside. Give it a poke to check for doneness. Serve with pan juices, garnished with mint.

# Oven-Steamed Fish with Ginger-Scallion Sauce

*Any filet o'fish will do. Serve this dish with rice to soak up all the juice.*

1 pound filet o' fish (I like cod or
  ocean catfish, Chilean sea bass,
  salmon, sole, or shellfish)
1 tablespoon or more olive oil
1 1/4 cup white wine, sake, or
  champagne
1 1/2 tablespoons, more or less, soy sauce
1 tablespoon fresh ginger, minced
1 bunch scallions (some green
  trimmed off ), quartered
  lengthwise

Preheat oven to 400°F.

In a small bowl, combine the oil, wine, soy sauce, and ginger. Put the fish in a baking dish and pour the sauce over it. Drape the scallions over the fish and cover the baking dish with tin foil.

Bake in preheated oven for 12 to 20 minutes, depending on the thickness of the fish. The fish is done when it *just* starts to flake apart with a fork.

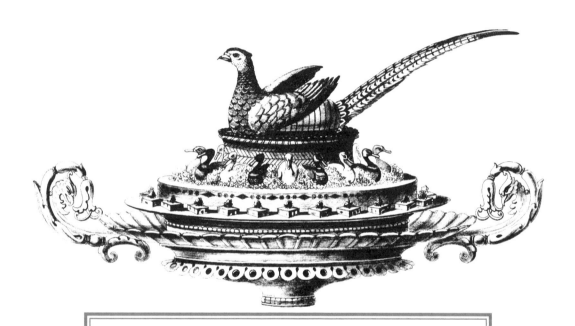

# POULTRY

# Sage Balsamic Chicken

*This may be the perfect marriage. For a change of herb, try using fresh thyme or oregano.*

1 tablespoon or more olive oil
2 tablespoons balsamic vinegar
1 teaspoon grated orange peel
1 tablespoon coarsely chopped fresh
　sage leaves
Salt and pepper to taste
1 pound boneless chicken thighs

Combine the oil, vinegar, and seasonings to make a marinade and let the chicken sit in it for 2 to 24 hours. Preheat oven to 400°F and bake chicken in preheated oven for about 25 minutes. Instead of baked, chicken may be broiled for 10 to 12 minutes, or grilled for 5 to 7 minutes on each side.

*A marinade creates instant variety and can be as simple as bottled salad dressing. Pour Italian dressing over chicken (fish or vegetables), let it sit for few a hours, cook it, and you've got chicken Italian style. Really. All the components of a marinade are in a salad dressing—oil for richness and browning; acid (citrus, vinegar, or wine) for tenderizing and tang; and seasonings (salt, pepper, garlic, herbs, and spices, etc.) to round out flavor. Try improvising your own marinade using this formula. It's a lot of fun and I know you can do it.*

# Green Green Chicken

*This recipe has its feet in two continents—one part Japanese, one part continental. Try the marinade with chicken, or try it with turkey, scallops, or a hearty fish.*

1 bunch cilantro leaves
1 jalapeño pepper, seeded and
   chopped
1 $^1/_2$ teaspoons Dijon mustard
1 tablespoon soy sauce
2 tablespoons freshly squeezed lime
   juice
2 tablespoons olive oil
2 cloves garlic, chopped
1 pound boneless chicken thighs

Puree all ingredients (except chicken) in a food processor to make a marinade. Marinate the chicken for 2 to 24 hours and bake in oven preheated to 400°F for 25 to 30 minutes.

*Marco Polo was the original fusion-meister. He traveled to the Orient, brought back noodles, coupled them with regional Italian ingredients, and caused a sensation. This is the root of fusion cuisine. It can be a beautiful sharing of cultures or a half-baked menu item. Adding ginger to beurre blanc does not a pleasing fusion make.*

# Jerk Chicken

*My version of the famous Jamaican spice rub works well with chicken, but a hearty fish such as shark or shellfish can also be used. This recipe makes enough for a pound of flesh.*

1 lime, zest and juice
2 tablespoons olive oil
1 tablespoon soy sauce
1 onion, finely chopped
1 jalapeño pepper (or more),
    seeded and finely chopped
2 cloves garlic, finely chopped
2 tablespoons allspice berries,
    ground up (I like to leave them a
    lime chunky)
1 teaspoon cinnamon powder
1 teaspoon thyme
1 teaspoon black pepper (freshly
    ground is best)
Pinch of salt

Buzz all ingredients together in a food processor to make a paste. Coat chicken (or fish) and marinate for 2 to 24 hours (only 30 minutes for fish). Grill, bake, or broil, turning as needed, until done.

*In Jamaica we would make stew by cooking down veggies and beans in coconut milk. No salt was added to the stew because we were cooking ital. Ital means "pure"— some Jamaicans (mainly Rastafarians) believe that salt constricts the body and spirit. They believe that if you put salt on a bird's tail it won't be able to fly and that a person who never ate salt could fly— spiritually and physically. I have a dilemma every time I pick up the salt shaker. To fly or not to fly. . . . I like my food salted, too bad it prevents liftoff.*

# Orange Cornish Game Hens

*Cornish game hens are fun to serve. A little bird for each guest.*

2 tablespoons olive oil

$^1/_4$ cup orange juice concentrate

2 tablespoons soy sauce

2 tablespoons orange marmalade

1 tablespoon chopped fresh
    rosemary leaf (or 1 teaspoon
    dry)

Freshly ground black pepper to
    taste

2 Cornish game hens, whole or split

Combine all the ingredients (except the hens) to make a marinade, pour it over the birdies, and let them soak it up for at least 2 hours (preferably overnight). To cook whole birds, preheat oven to 375°F and bake for 45 to 55 minutes. To cook split birds, grill for 10 to 12 minutes on each side.

# Mongolian BBQ

*A metal sheet over an open fire was the cookery of choice for the nomadic Mongolians. Try a nonstick cookie sheet over 2 burners to adapt today's home fires for this dish, which serves 4 to 6. (Electric burners will work but be careful of burning.) For variety, substitute other meats and vegetables.*

### For the marinade:

$3/4$ *cup soy sauce*
*2 cups water or stock*
*12 peppercorns, crushed*
*4 whole-star anise, crushed*
*3 cloves garlic, crushed*
$1/2$ *cup sake*
*2 teaspoons sweetener*
*1 bunch cilantro leaves, chopped*
*1 bunch scallions, chopped*

### For the rest:

*2 pounds boneless chicken thighs*
*1 pound assorted seafood (optional)*
*2 bunches watercress, left in whole*
  *sprigs*
*1 pound bean sprouts*
*1 pound carrots*
*Vegetable oil (or peanut or canola),*
  *for sautéing*

Combine marinade ingredients and set aside.

Put the chicken thighs in the freezer until slightly frozen, about 30 minutes.

Clean the vegetables and set aside. Cut the carrots into matchsticks.

Slice the partially frozen chicken very thin.

Set the cookie sheet over the burners (or use a wok, griddle, or large frying pan), oil well, and light up at moderate heat. Let your guests dip any combination of chicken (or other meat), veggies, and seafood if desired into the marinade, then place on the oiled metal sheet and cook to doneness (it only takes a few minutes). Serve with Mongolian Flatbread (p. 67) and white rice.

# Poulet à la Diàble

*A devilishly tangy marinade for chicken or hearty fish.*

1 pound boneless chicken
1 tablespoon olive oil
2 bay leaves, crumbled
2 cloves garlic, minced
$1/2$ cup white wine
2 teaspoons Dijon mustard
6 or 7 dashes Tabasco sauce (or
   more to taste)
Salt and pepper to taste

Combine all the ingredients (except the chicken if you please) to make a marinade and marinate the chicken for 2 to 12 hours.

Grill or broil marinated chicken for a few minutes on each side until charred but still juicy.

*The source of "heat" in any dish comes from hot peppers. When I lived in Jamaica we always added a pepper to the pot. There the peppers grew on little treelike bushes. The chickens would jump up, necks outstretched, and pluck these extremely hot peppers off their branches and munch away. They have a saying in Jamaica, "who feels it knows it." I guess chickens don't know it. Just after sundown, our whole family of chickens lined up on a tree branch and went to sleep. It's an image I can't shake.*

# Green Curry Chicken

*You have to indulge once in a while. Without the coconut milk this dish doesn't work, so enjoy.*

1 $\frac{1}{2}$ tablespoons green curry paste
   (to make your own, see below)
1 14-ounce can coconut milk
1 pound boneless chicken thighs,
   each thigh cut into quarters
1 onion, sliced thin
1 $\frac{1}{2}$ tablespoons or more fish sauce to
   taste
1 tablespoon or more sweetener to
   taste
1 large handful green beans
1 large red bell pepper, sliced
1 eggplant, prebaked (40 minutes
   at 400°F) or microwaved (5
   minutes)
1 cup fresh pineapple chunks
   (canned if you must)
Fresh basil leaves as garnish

In a wok or large frying pan, stir and fry the curry paste with 2 tablespoons of the coconut milk, blending them together, over high heat for 1 or 2 minutes (*brown,* don't burn). Add the chicken and the onion and stir-fry for a few more minutes (chicken should begin to brown). Add the rest of the coconut milk, the fish sauce, the sweetener, the green beans, the pepper, and the eggplant and bring to a low boil. Lower the heat to a simmer, add the pineapple, and cook until the chicken is tender.

Check for seasoning and serve hot garnished with basil leaves over white rice.

# TIP

*Boneless chicken thighs are about half the price of boneless breasts. They're juicier and more flavorful too. You can use thighs for any boneless chicken recipe and they'll taste great even if you overcook them.*

# Green Curry Paste

*In case green curry paste is not available in your neighborhood, here's an easy recipe.*

5 hot green chili peppers (serrano
    or jalapeño), chopped
2 stalks lemongrass (or 4 dried
slices lemon, chopped
5 cloves garlic, chopped
1 teaspoon galingale powder,
    optional
$^1/_2$ teaspoon salt

Puree all ingredients in a food processor to make a thick, green paste.

*There are only so many ways to cook and most cultures use them all. Bake, broil, fry, steam, boil, sauté—it's the same in any language. The difference is in the spices and flavorings each region uses. Making a few dishes of a particular cuisine will familiarize you with a region's characteristic flavors. After that, it's all method. If you can cook Italian, you can cook Chinese, and if there's someone out there I can't teach to make a Thai curry, I'll eat my car (not a compact). It's that fundamental.*

# Chicken à la Creole

*All day flavor in less than an hour. You can't beat it.*

1 tablespoon olive oil
1½ to 2 pounds boneless chicken
    thighs
1 large onion, chopped
2 green bell peppers, chopped
2 cloves garlic, minced
2 tablespoons white flour
4 large tomatoes, chopped
2 bay leaves
1 teaspoon thyme
Salt and pepper to taste
½ cup chicken stock
Chopped parsley

Heat the oil over high heat in a wok or large frying pan and sauté the chicken with the onion and the peppers. When the chicken begins to brown, add the garlic and continue to cook for ½ minute. Add the flour to the pan and stir and fry until well blended, 2 or 3 minutes. Add the tomatoes, bay leaves, thyme, salt and pepper, and the stock and bring to a boil. Lower the heat to just simmering and cook for 15 to 20 minutes, stirring occasionally to prevent sticking (watch for bottom-sticking). Serve over rice, garnished with chopped parsley.

# Shish Taouk

*The real name for Middle Eastern shish kebab. Simple spicing adds mucho flavor.*

Juice of 1 lemon
2 tablespoons olive oil
1 teaspoon paprika
1 teaspoon thyme
Salt and pepper to taste
1 pound boneless chicken, cut into
    chunks
1 large onion, cut into bite-sized
    chunks
2 bell peppers, cut into bite-sized
    chunks

Mix the lemon juice with the oil, paprika, thyme, and salt and pepper. Add the chicken and vegetables and let it all sit for at least 2 hours (preferably overnight).

Skewer chunks and broil or grill to doneness.

*Being broke in London taught me how to cook; here's the recipe: food-loving hungry lad with very little funds. I'd go down to the corner store, buy a few bits and pieces, and ask the Pakistani shopkeeper how to prepare it. Sometimes he'd lay some spices on me. I learned to improvise because I had to. This lad still likes to eat, and those meals were especially good. I'm not suggesting that you recreate this condition—it's bleak—but necessity is the mother of invention.*

# Grilled Chicken, Yucatan Style

*Another zinger for the grill.*

1 fryer chicken, cut into parts
1 cup fresh orange juice
2 tablespoons olive oil
1 teaspoon orange zest
4 cloves garlic, chopped
$1/2$ teaspoon thyme
$1/2$ teaspoon oregano
$1/2$ teaspoon marjoram
4 bay leaves, crumbled
Salt and pepper to taste

Combine all ingredients and marinate overnight. Grill over moderate heat, turning a few times, to desired doneness.

# TIP

*If you'd like to get to know the taste of a particular herb, make a dish that's chock-full of it. For example, take a Cornish game hen, stuff it with a handful of fresh sage, and roast it in the oven.*

# Pecan-Lime Chicken

*The combination of lime juice, fragrant pecans, and doughy bread gives this dish its unique texture and flavor.*

$1/4$ cup lime juice

2 tablespoons olive oil

$1/2$ cup pecans

2 thick slices of French bread,
  cut into small cubes

1 16-ounce can peeled tomatoes

Salt and pepper to taste

1 pound boneless chicken (thighs
  are recommended)

Blend all ingredients (except chicken) in a food processor to a chunky consistency, pour it over the chicken in a baking dish, and refrigerate. After a few hours (or as long as you like) bake the chicken in the marinade, in oven preheated to 400°F, for 20 to 25 minutes.

*So what if I'm an ovo-lacto, pseudo-macro, poultry-eatin' son of a sea cook. I'm an omnivore and that means choices. People like to have a label to make it easier to invite you over for dinner. I'm going to send postcards listing everything I eat and don't eat to a mailing list of potential dinner hosts and wait for the phone to ring.... I'm still waiting.*

# Thai Citrus-Grilled Chicken

*Coriander, aka cilantro, aka Chinese parsley—it's all the same plant.*

1 pound boneless chicken, in whole parts or cut into small pieces for skewering

1 bunch fresh coriander root, the white and a little green, chopped

$^1/_2$ teaspoon black pepper

1 tablespoon Thai fish sauce

$^1/_4$ cup coconut milk (or more)

$^1/_2$ teaspoon turmeric

2 teaspoons sweetener

Juice of 1 orange

Juice of 1 lime

4 to 6 cloves garlic, chopped

Place the coriander root, pepper, fish sauce, coconut milk, turmeric, sweetener, citrus, and garlic in a food processor and puree to use as a marinade. Submerge the chicken in the marinade and refrigerate for 2 to 24 hours. Whenever you're ready, grill it over high heat, turning chicken, till you get it right.

# Fajitas

*Fajita means "skirt steak" in spanish but has come to mean something else in the States. A sort of Mexican stir-fry*—es bueno.

**For the marinade:**

*2 tablespoons olive oil*

*Juice of 2 limes*

*2 tablespoons soy sauce*

*2 teaspoons Worcestershire sauce*

*1 teaspoon oregano*

*2 cloves garlic, minced*

*2 teaspoons sweetener*

*Pinch of paprika*

*Salt and pepper to taste*

**The stuff to marinate (just veggies is good too):**

*1 pound sliced boneless chicken thighs or 1 pound cut up seafood (or combo of both)*

*1 large Spanish onion, sliced thin*

*2 bell peppers (red or yellow are nice), sliced thin*

*Other veggies as desired (mushroom, broccoli, zucchini, tomatoes, whatever)*

Combine the marinade ingredients, add the stuff, and marinate for 1 to 24 hours. (If using seafood, marinate for only 20 minutes or less and keep it separate if combining with chicken because it takes less time to cook).

Heat a cast-iron skillet or a wok over medium-high heat and add some olive oil. Pick the veggies and poultry out of the marinade and toss them into the pan. Hear the sizzle. Stir and fry. (As the pan gets dry, add some of the marinade. By the time the chicken and veggies are done, you should have added all the remaining marinade.)

Put some hot pads on the table to set the pan on and serve family style. For real Mexican flair, try serving with warmed flour tortillas—take a tortilla and fill with a combo of all this stuff—along with salsa, refried or black beans, plain nonfat yogurt, guacamole, rice, and salad on the side: *Felicidads!*

# Chicken Picatta

*Make this dish with chicken, turkey, or seafood (maybe even tofu). Can't miss if you like lemon.*
*Potato flour gives it a nice, slightly doughy texture. Serve over a small amount of pasta to pick up*
*the pan juices.*

1 pound boneless chicken thighs or
   breast
Salt and pepper to taste
Potato flour or white flour
2 tablespoons, more or less, olive oil
$^1/_4$ cup lemon juice
2 tablespoons chopped parsley

Cut the chicken into ring-finger-sized strips or slice into medallions. Season with salt and pepper and dredge in potato flour to coat.

In a nonstick frying pan, heat the olive oil moderately and add the dredged chicken (spread 'em out—no pileups). Turn the chicken when it's nice and golden brown and continue to cook. When the chicken is firm to the touch, turn off the heat and add the lemon juice and the parsley. Toss and serve immediately.

# Chicken, Onion, and Apple

*A New England home-style meal in minutes. The sauce is delicious. This recipe also works well with turkey.*

4 small boneless chicken thighs (or
  1 large boneless turkey thigh)
Salt and pepper to taste
1 tablespoon olive oil
1 apple, cored and sliced into $1/4$-inch-
  thick rounds
1 onion, sliced into $1/4$-inch-thick
  rounds
$1/2$ cup white wine (I like Zinfandel
  but whatever you're drinking is
  okay)

Season chicken or turkey with salt and pepper (if using turkey, cut thigh into 4 equal parts not more than $1^1/_2$ inches thick). Heat the oil over medium-high heat in a large frying pan and place the meat in the pan. Put a slice of apple and then a slice of onion on each piece of poultry and cover the pan. Cook for 7 to 8 minutes, until well browned (lift it a little and have a look at the underside).

Uncover the pan (and leave uncovered from here on out) and turn the meat so the onion is on the bottom, the apple in the middle, and the poultry on top. Continue to cook for about 5 to 7 minutes (depending on the thickness of the pieces; check for firmness). Add the wine to the pan and cook until it is reduced by almost half. Flip out onto plates and serve, drizzled with or surrounded by pan juices.

# Suki Sake

*It's fun to cook this dish at table: Use a hot plate or an Oriental-style gas burner. This recipe serves 2 as an entree or 4 as a side dish.*

1 pound boneless chicken thighs, cut
    into thin strips
2 carrots, cut at an angle into
    medium slices
6 scallion bottoms (white and a little
    green)
1 zuchinni, cut into thick slices
1 cup broccoli florets
1 red pepper, cut into thick slices
$^1/_2$ cup sake
2 teaspoons dry sweetener
4 tablespoons low-sodium soy sauce
    (or less to taste)
2 cups chicken stock
6 slices ginger, cut into matchsticks
About 2 cups cooked Chinese-style
    noodles or udon

Arrange the chicken, the vegetables, and the noodles (shell-fish will work too, but with shellfish cut the vegetables into smaller pieces so that everything will have a similar cooking time) in groups—a sort of mini mosaic—in a large cast-iron skillet or a wok. Combine the liquid ingredients and the ginger and pour over the chicken and veggies. (You can do this in advance and let it marinate for a while or just go ahead and cook it.) Cook over medium heat (at table or on the stove) until it comes to a rolling boil. Reduce heat to a simmer and continue to cook for about 10 minutes. Check the chicken for doneness—it should be firm. You might have to turn it if it's piled up.

When the chicken is ready, it's time to eat. Give everyone a bowl and dig in right from the skillet.

# Five-Spice Turkey Tenders

*The marinade in this dish may be used for any type of poultry. If you can't find 5-spice powder use equal amounts of cinnamon, cloves, aniseed, and nutmeg.*

1 pound turkey tender (ask for it at the meat counter—it's the underside of the breast)
2 tablespoons rice wine or sherry
1 tablespoon dark sesame oil
1 tablespoon fresh ginger, minced
1 clove garlic, chopped fine
1 teaspoon five-spice powder
1 $^1/_2$ tablespoons soy sauce
$^1/_2$ teaspoon orange zest
Pinch of black pepper

Combine all ingredients in a bowl and marinate for 2 to 4 hours. Grill or broil whole tender(s) for 7 to 10 minutes on each side or cut into slices and stir-fry.

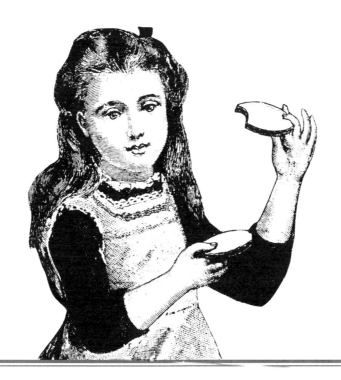

# DESSERTS

# Grilled-Pineapple Skewers

*A juicy summer dessert without much work. Fire makes my fronded friend more succulent.*

*Fresh pineapple chunks*
*Molasses*
*Wooden skewers*

Skewer chunks of pineapple, brush with molasses, and grill over moderate heat. Let those babies brown and caramelize to bring out the natural sugars: you'll be glad you did!

# TIP

*An organized kitchen is a chef's best friend. If you use something a lot, keep it out. Keeping the things you use near the stove will get you in and out of the kitchen more quickly and lead you there more often.*

# Almond Cake with Strawberry Sauce

*I made this one evening for my Valentine. We didn't get to it that night, but it was great the next day.*

**For the almond cake:**
*I cup vanilla soy milk (or milk)*
*I cup apple juice*
*¹/₂ cup applesauce*
*2 tablespoons corn oil*
*I teaspoon almond extract, optional*
*I cup toasted slivered almonds*
*I cup whole wheat (or white) pastry flour*
*I cup unbleached white flour*
*I tablespoon baking powder*
*Dash of salt*

Preheat oven to 350°F.

Buzz the almonds in a food processor to a fine consistency and combine with the remaining dry ingredients—flours, baking powder, and salt—in a large bowl and whisk together. In a separate bowl, combine all the wet ingredients, add them to the dry, and mix. Do not overmix.

Pour batter into a greased pie pan (heart-shaped if you've got one) and bake in preheated oven for 35 to 40 minutes, until nicely browned on top.

**For the strawberry sauce:**
*I package frozen strawberries*
*¹/₂ cup apple juice*
*Juice of ¹/₂ lemon*
*I tablespoon cornstarch*

Combine strawberries, apple juice, and lemon juice in a saucepan and bring to a boil. Lower the heat and simmer for about 10 minutes.

Dilute the cornstarch in a few tablespoons of juice or water, stir into the strawberry mixture, and turn off the heat. Puree in a food processor and serve warm, drizzled over slices of fresh baked almond cake, or follow the presentation suggested below.

**Presentation:**
Cut the cake into 2 thin layers. Use the sauce as a middle layer and over the top. For a fancy presentation, fill a cleaned-out ketchup or other squeeze bottle with nonfat yogurt (flavor of choice) and squirt a design over the cake.

# Strawberry Sorbet

*Easy to make, fun to serve. Top with strawberry sauce (p. 125) for a strawberry overdose (of a good thing).*

1 quart full-flavored strawberries
$^1/_2$ cup frozen apple juice concentrate
2 tablespoons lemon juice

Puree all ingredients in a food processor, pour into a bowl, cover, and freeze for 3 or 4 hours.

Remove the bowl from the freezer about every 45 minutes and puree again for a smooth consistency. Let the sorbet sit out at room temperature for 15 minutes or so before serving.

# TIP

*Frozen apple juice concentrate and orange juice concentrate (that stuff in paper cans that you add water to to make juice) are great for baking and marinades. They have an intensely sweet and fruity flavor without refined sugar.*

# Mount Fuji Apple Bake

*I know it's a little weird but try it anyway.*

4 apples, cored and cut into long thin
   slices
1 tablespoon or more fresh ginger,
   peeled and cut into very thin
   matchsticks
Juice of 2 oranges
2 tablespoons honey or other
   sweetener
1 tablespoon dark sesame oil
1 tablespoon sesame seeds

Preheat oven to 350°F.

Mix the apple slices with the ginger and make a mountain of them in the center of a Pyrex pie plate. Pour the orange juice over the ginger-apple mountain, drizzle with honey and oil, and sprinkle with sesame seeds.

Bake in preheated oven for 45 minutes.

# Grilled Bananas with Dark Rum

*If a grill isn't handy, fry the bananas in a pan. A fitting end to an Oriental meal . . . or a romantic breakfast in bed.*

4 firm bananas, sliced in half
   lengthwise
1 shot of dark rum
2 tablespoons molasses
$1/2$ teaspoon cinnamon
$1/4$ teaspoon nutmeg
1 tablespoon corn oil
1 teaspoon vanilla extract

Combine all ingredients and marinate at room temperature for 2 hours or more. Grill (or fry in corn oil) until browned. Serve hot, topped with frozen yogurt if desired.

# Strawberries Modena

*Serve this simple dessert in a martini glass for a touch of class.*

1 pint strawberries
1 tablespoon orange juice
1 teaspoon (or a little more)
   balsamic vinegar
Orange zest, as garnish

Gently toss the strawberries with the orange juice and the vinegar. Serve in individual portions garnished with orange zest.

# Oranges with Mint

*Contrasting flavors that refresh. Enjoy.*

4 large temple (or other) oranges,
   peeled, cut into $^1/_2$-inch slices
1 tablespoon orange liqueur
2 tablespoons chopped fresh mint
   leaves

Arrange the orange slices on a platter, drizzle with orange liqueur, and garnish with chopped mint leaves.

# Pineapple in White Wine

*Dry white wine brings out the tang of the noble pineapple. Crisp, refreshing, even elegant.*

1 ripe pineapple, peeled, cored,
   quartered lengthwise, and cut
   into thin slices
1 cup dry white wine
2 teaspoons, more or less,
   sweetener
Fresh mint leaves, chopped, as
   garnish

Arrange the pineapple slices in a shallow bowl or deep platter, pour the wine over them, sprinkle or drizzle with sweetener, and garnish with chopped fresh mint leaves. That's it!

## TIP

*A pineapple is one of nature's perfect packages. It's beautiful (in a prehistoric, scaly, frondy kind of way) and the succulent yellow flesh has a phenomenal balance of sweet and sour flavors. A pineapple is an elegant, distinct, and exotic dessert all by itself. The trick is picking a ripe one. The best test is to turn one over and smell its bottom. It should smell like canned pineapple perfume.*

# Fresh Fruit Marsala

*Have fun with fresh fruit and a little booze.*

$^1/_2$ cup marsala wine
Juice of 2 oranges
2 tablespoons or more sweetener
1 teaspoon cinnamon
Pinch of nutmeg
4 cups mixed fresh fruit (apples,
   pears, peaches, etc.), sliced thin
1 package frozen berries with syrup

In a wok or large frying pan, combine the wine, orange juice, sweetener, and spices over medium heat and bring to a simmer. Add the fruit, turn off the heat, and let sit for an hour or more. Reheat gently to serve hot (alone or as a topping for vanilla frozen yogurt) or serve cold with a dollop of plain yogurt.

*I worked at a juice bar in L.A. called "I Love Juicy." It was owned by an ex-cab driver from Brooklyn who was hell-bent for health. We made ice cream out of frozen fruit and some killer, no-bake tropical fruit pies. I had one too many shots of wheatgrass one night and decided to retire from the juicy business. The owner, whose motto was "Ask not what juicy can do for you, but what you can do for juicy," considered me a defector at this point and called the cops. He told them there was a disturbance at I Love Juicy, and then he didn't want to pay me the money he owed me and pretended to come at me with a prep knife. I wonder if he was crazy before he started eating that stuff?*

# Figs, Sherry, and Vanilla

*A creamy blend of rich flavors, simple and exotic—the perfect finale to a paella feast.*

$^1/_2$ pound dried figs

2 cups cream sherry (or more as needed)

1 whole vanilla bean, split lengthwise

Place the figs and the split vanilla bean in a saucepan and cover with sherry. Bring to a boil and reduce the heat to a low simmer. Simmer the figs for 30 to 40 minutes, adding extra sherry if the figs absorb all the liquid, until soft and tender to the touch. Serve hot or cold, alone or over vanilla frozen yogurt.

# Fruit Cobbler

*This fruit-sweetened dessert warms body and soul and fills your home with an aroma that will keep everybody in the kitchen.*

3 cups sliced or diced apples (or peaches or pears, or I quart whole blueberries, etc.)

2 cups apple juice (or other fruit juice)

I tablespoon white flour

2 teaspoons cinnamon (or apple pie spice, cloves, nutmeg, ginger, etc.)

I ¹/₂ cups rolled oats

¹/₂ cup pastry flour (or toasted wheat germ)

2 tablespoons or more corn oil

¹/₂ cup whole walnuts

Preheat oven to 350°F.

Dice the apples (or peaches or pears) into I-inch squares or cut into thin slices. Place in a large pie plate.

Reserve 2 tablespoons of the fruit juice. Mix the remaining fruit juice with the I tablespoon of white flour and I teaspoon of the cinnamon and pour over the fruit.

In a separate bowl, mix the oats, the pastry flour, the remaining teaspoon of cinnamon, the oil, and the 2 tablespoons reserved fruit juice and crumble together with your hands to work in the oil.

Sprinkle the oat mixture over the fruit and top with the nuts.

Bake in preheated oven until well browned, about 50 to 60 minutes.

*"Organic" is the designer food label of the '90s. Designer consciousness began in the '60s with Pierre Cardin. He was the first to actually use his name to add value to whatever he was selling. Since then, well, you know the story, everybody wants a label. My first recollection of designer food was at Boston University in the late '70s. My roommate was from New York and had to have Pepperidge Farm chocolate chip cookies and Haagen-Dāzs chocolate ice cream (along with an herbal supplement) nightly or he couldn't sleep. He said that "H.D. ice cream comes in a hard, frozen state for shipping purposes, but everyone in New York knows that you have to leave it out at room temperature for twenty minutes before consumption." I was impressed.*

# Caramel Corn

*I love this stuff. The secret to the perfect caramel corn is watching it very closely in the last minutes of cooking. Rice syrup is available in natural food stores and it's not as sweet as honey or corn syrup. Rent a movie. Enjoy.*

$^1/_2$ cup popcorn

1 tablespoon corn oil (unrefined if you've got it), optional

Salt to taste

8 to 10 ounces rice syrup

Pecans (or peanuts)

Preheat oven to 375°F.

Use the oil to pop the corn in the microwave or to cook it conventionally or air-pop it without oil if desired. Put the popped corn in a large baking dish (don't pile it up too much) and sprinkle with salt (I like to use a bit of salt here because I like the contrast of sweet and salt). Liberally drizzle the rice syrup over the popcorn and lay the nuts (as many or as few as you like) on top.

Bake in preheated oven for about 20 minutes. When the syrup starts to brown, watch it very closely. When it seems as dark as it can get without burning, it's done. Take it out of the oven and use a wooden spoon or a spatula to scrape it into a large bowl. For maximum crunch, let it cool before digging in.

# Quick Breads and Muffins

*Use the basic recipe to create endless variations (see suggested variations at right). This recipe makes 6 muffins or 1 loaf of bread. There's no substitute for fresh baked muffins and breads so give this recipe a try.*

## Dry ingredients:

1 cup unbleached white flour
1 cup pastry flour (preferably whole wheat)
2$^1/_2$ teaspoons baking powder
Large pinch of salt
1 teaspoon cinnamon or other
    sweet spices

## Wet ingredients:

1 egg (or 2 egg whites)
$^1/_2$ cup apple juice, or $^1/_2$ cup frozen
    apple juice concentrate, thawed,
      if you like a more intense fruit flavor
$^1/_2$ cup soy milk or milk
2 tablespoons corn oil (optional)
$^1/_4$ cup sweetener, more or less
    (optional)

Preheat the oven to 350°F.

In a large bowl, whisk together all the dry ingredients.

In a separate bowl, whisk together all the wet ingredients and use a rubber spatula or wooden spoon to mix into the dry just enough to blend. Do not overmix. To test consistency, hold the spatula or spoon over the bowl with a dollop of batter on it. The batter should fall off (glop) into the bowl after a second or so. If it doesn't fall, it's too dry, so add a little liquid (juice or milk). If it falls too fast, add a little flour. (If desired, this is the time to add any additional ingredients—such as bananas, nuts, berries, etc. See suggestions at right.)

Spoon batter into greased bread pan, pie plate, or muffin tins and bake: 35 to 40 minutes for a loaf pan, 25 to 30 minutes for a pie plate, or 15 to 20 minutes for muffins.

 **TIP**

*When baking quick breads and muffins, the best way to test for doneness is to gently press the center with your finger. If they're leavened, the center should slowly rise back.*

**Variations:**

- For **Banana Bread** add I large mashed banana and I teaspoon of vanilla and top with walnuts.
- For **Blueberry Muffins** add I cup of fresh or frozen blueberries.
- For **Blueberry Streusel Muffins** top blueberry muffins (above) with $^1/_2$ cup walnuts sautéed in 2 tablespoons corn or other vegetable oil with I teaspoon cinnamon and 2 tablespoons sweetener *before baking*.
- For **Bran Muffins** add $^1/_2$ cup wheat bran, $^1/_2$ cup raisins, and an additional $^1/_3$ cup frozen apple juice concentrate, thawed.
- For **Crunchy Granola Muffins** add $^3/_4$ cup prepared granola and 2 tablespoons peanut butter and top with granola and an additional $^1/_4$ cup apple juice.
- For **Orange Poppy-Seed Muffins** use orange juice concentrate instead of apple and add ($^1/_3$ cup poppy seeds.
- For **Coconut Date Bread** use $^1/_2$ cup coconut milk and $^1/_4$ cup thawed frozen orange juice concentrate (in place of milk and apple juice) for liquid ingredients, add $^1/_2$ cup chopped dates, and top with shredded coconut.

# Every Day Apple Pie

*Any kind of apples—except red delicious and mushy Macs—will do. I like this à la mode with a drizzle of chocolate sauce.*

**For the crust:**

2 cups rolled oats
1 cup wheat germ, toasted
$1/2$ cup slivered almonds, toasted
2 tablespoons corn oil
$1/2$ cup apple juice concentrate
   (you know, the frozen stuff in the
   can before you add water to it),
   thawed, or other liquid sweetener
$1/2$ teaspoon cinnamon

Preheat oven to 350°F.

Buzz all ingredients in a food processor until fairly fine but still granular. Reserve about 1 cup of the crust mix for a crumble topping. Press remaining crust mixture into a greased pie pan (as thinly as possible with no pan peeking through) and bake in preheated oven for 15 minutes. Remove baked crust and let it cool before filling. Leave the oven on.

**Or, for a really easy crust:**

4 cups granola (store-bought)
2 tablespoons corn oil
3 tablespoons juice, any kind

Preheat oven to 350°F.

Buzz all ingredients in a food processor and prepare as above.

**For the pie filling:**

6 apples, peeled if desired, cored, and
   sliced thin

2 tablespoons dry sweetener (brown
   sugar, Sucanat, or other)

2 tablespoons juice (concentrate or
   other)

1 heaping tablespoon white flour

$^1/_2$ teaspoon or more cinnamon or apple
   pie spice mix

In a large bowl, combine all ingredients, mix well, and pour into the prebaked pie shell. Crumble reserved crust mixture over the whole affair and bake at 350°F for 50 minutes. Serve with your favorite frozen dessert.

*Once I had a hot fudge sundae that was completely nondairy, was low in fat, and contained no refined sugar. It was so good I had another (why not, it's health food). You can get almost any nostalgia food in a health-food version these days—tofu hot dogs, sugar-free ketchup, turkey bacon, vegetarian chili, veggie burgers, natural honey-frosted flakes, malt-sweetened chocolate balls, and even organic M&M's. When I tell people about my sundae they ask me if it was as good as the original. I tell them, "Probably not, but after you've forgotten what the original tastes like, it's pretty damn good."*

# Shortcut Guide to Marinades and Quick Sauces

A marinade creates instant variety and is made up of three basic components—oil for richness and browning; acid (vinegar, wine, citrus juice) for tenderizing and tang; and seasonings to round out and define flavor.

Listed below are a variety of delicious and diverse approaches to the same solution—the marvelous marinade. For any of these suggestions, simply combine all the ingredients, marinate your fishes—for no more than 20 to 30 minutes (any longer and fish can get too tough)—or your chicken—for up to 24 hours—in an oven-safe dish, and then bake, broil, or grill to desired doneness.

A marinade can easily become a sauce: Dilute 1 tablespoon of flour in $1/4$ cup of water and add to the marinade to create a sauce while baking. The marinade will mix with the pan juices for the perfect saucy marriage. Each of the following recipes makes enough marinade for 1 pound of whatever. Have fun with any or all of them and feel free to add, subtract, or otherwise personalize the recipes.

### Mongolian BBQ

2 tablespoons soy sauce, 3 tablespoons rice wine, 1 tablespoon vegetable oil, 2 cloves minced garlic, 1 teaspoon sweetener, 1 tablespoon chopped cilantro leaves, 1 chopped scallion, black pepper, $1/2$ teaspoon aniseed or 2 crushed whole aniseed stars

### Balsamic Vinegar and Sage

2 tablespoons or less olive oil, 2 to 3 tablespoons balsamic vinegar, $^1/_2$ teaspoon orange peel, 1 tablespoon chopped fresh sage leaves (or 1 teaspoon dry), salt and pepper

### Fajita-Style

1 tablespoon soy sauce, 1 tablespoon olive oil, 2 tablespoons lime juice, 1 teaspoon Worcestershire sauce, $^1/_2$ teaspoon oregano, 1 or 2 cloves minced garlic, salt and black pepper, pinch paprika, 1 teaspoon sweetener, a gulp of white wine (optional)

### Southwestern BBQ

1 tablespoon olive oil, $^1/_4$ cup canned crushed pineapple with juice, 2 tablespoons tomato paste, 1 tablespoon molasses (or 2 teaspoons brown sugar), 1 teaspoon chili powder, $^1/_2$ teaspoon cumin, 1 teaspoon prepared mustard, Tabasco sauce to taste, salt and pepper

### Middle Eastern

2 tablespoons or less olive oil, 3 to 4 tablespoons lemon juice, 2 cloves chopped garlic, $^1/_2$ teaspoon paprika, $^1/_2$ teaspoon thyme, $^1/_2$ chopped onion, salt and pepper

### Chinese Five-Spice

1 tablespoon sesame or peanut oil, 2 tablespoons rice wine or sherry, $1^1/_2$ tablespoons soy sauce, 4 slices fresh ginger, 1 clove chopped garlic, 1 teaspoon sweetener, 1 teaspoon five-spice powder, $^1/_4$ teaspoon orange zest, black pepper

### French Herbal

1 tablespoon or more olive oil, $^1/_4$ cup red wine, 1 tablespoon tomato paste, 1 tablespoon fresh rosemary leaves (or 1 teaspoon dry), 1 tablespoon fresh thyme leaves (or 1 teaspoon dry), 1 crushed bay leaf, 1 clove chopped garlic, salt and pepper

### Thai Citrus

2 tablespoons coconut milk, 1 tablespoon fish sauce, $^1/_4$ cup orange juice, 2 cloves garlic, minced, 1 tablespoon minced cilantro root, $^1/_2$ teaspoon turmeric, 1 teaspoon sweetener, black pepper

### Yucatan

1 to 2 tablespoons olive oil, $^1/_4$ cup orange juice, 1 tablespoon lime juice, 3 or 4 cloves garlic, minced, $^1/_2$ teaspoon orange zest, $^1/_2$ teaspoon thyme, $^1/_2$ teaspoon oregano, $^1/_2$ teaspoon marjoram, 4 crushed bay leaves, salt and pepper

### Orange-Rosemary

2 tablespoons olive oil, $^1/_4$ cup orange juice, 2 tablespoons or less soy sauce, 2 tablespoons orange marmalade, 1 tablespoon fresh rosemary leaf (or 1 teaspoon dry), black pepper

### Diàble

1 tablespoon olive oil, $^1/_4$ cup white wine, 2 teaspoons prepared mustard, 2 cloves chopped garlic, 2 bay leaves, 6 or 7 dashes Tabasco, salt and pepper

## Orange-Ginger

$1/4$ cup orange juice, 1 teaspoon prepared mustard, 2 tablespoons olive oil, 1 tablespoon fresh minced ginger, salt and pepper

## Sherry-Shallot

2 tablespoons olive oil, 3 tablespoons sherry wine vinegar, 1 teaspoon Dijon mustard, 1 minced shallot, salt and pepper

## Mustard-Tarragon

2 tablespoons olive oil, $1/4$ cup white wine or champagne, 2 teaspoons prepared mustard, 1 tablespoon fresh chopped tarragon leaves (or 1 heaping teaspoon dry), salt and pepper

## Tandoori Style

3 tablespoons coconut milk (or yogurt), 1 tablespoon lime juice, 1 tablespoon fresh ginger, 2 cloves garlic, $1/2$ teaspoon orange zest, $1/2$ teaspoon paprika, 1 teaspoon curry powder, salt and pepper

# Index